PACIFIC PEDIATRIC CARDIOLOGY
50 W. Bellefontaine #405
Pasadena, California 91105

THE HEART OF A CHILD

The Heart of a Child

WHAT FAMILIES NEED TO KNOW
ABOUT HEART DISORDERS
IN CHILDREN

Catherine A. Neill, M.D.

Edward B. Clark, M.D.

Carleen Clark, R.N.

The Johns Hopkins University Press
Baltimore and London

Illustrations (unless noted otherwise) by Jacqueline Schaffer

Excerpt from "Bats" reprinted with permission of Macmillan Publishing
Company; from *The Bat-Poet,* by Randall Jarrell. Copyright © Macmillan
Publishing Company, 1963, 1964.

The Johns Hopkins University Press
701 West 40th Street
Baltimore, Maryland 21211-2190
The Johns Hopkins Press Ltd., London

Note to the reader. This book is not meant to substitute for medical care
of infants, children, or adults with heart problems, and treatment should
not be based solely on its contents. Instead, treatment must be developed
in a dialogue between the individual and his or her physician or between
the family and the child's physician. Our book has been written to help
with that dialogue.

Library of Congress Cataloging-in-Publication Data
Neill, Catherine A.
     The heart of a child : what families need to know about heart
disorders in children / Catherine A. Neill, Edward B. Clark, Carleen
Clark.
          p.   cm.
     Includes bibliographical references and index.
     ISBN 0-8018-4234-4 (hc : alk. paper)
     1. Congenital heart disease in children. 2. Heart—Diseases.
3. Children—Diseases.   I. Clark, Edward B.   II. Clark, Carleen.
III. Title.
     [DNLM: 1. Heart Defects, Congenital. 2. Heart Diseases—in
infancy & childhood.   WS 290 N411h]
RJ426.C64N45   1992
618.92 ' 12043—dc20
DNLM/DLC
for Library of Congress   92-25198

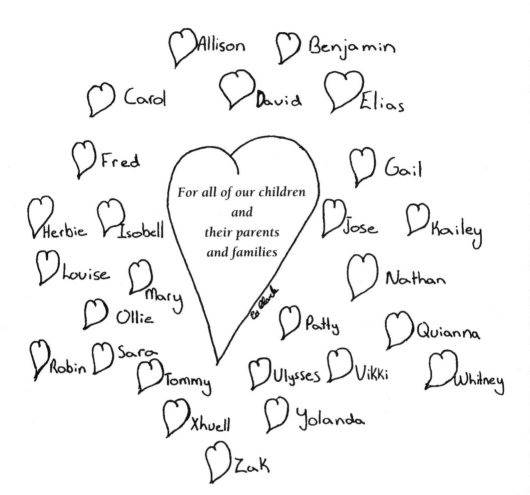

For all of our children and their parents and families

Courtesy Ed Clark, age 12

Contents

Illustrations

THE HEART OF A CHILD

The Heart of a Child

There is no more joyful sight than a child at play. The abundant energy, the swift, graceful movements, the sudden laugh all evoke a sense of the beauty and wonder of a vibrant young life. We take for granted the child's healthy circulation, the body's ability to provide oxygen to meet its demands.

It is easy to forget, when we see an energetic child at play, that not all children are born with healthy hearts. Many readers of this book have children who were born with heart defects; others are curious about different heart problems, such as heart murmurs. The main focus of this book is the heart of a child: what can be done to understand and treat a defect in a child's heart and how we can help a child who has a healthy heart keep it healthy. We now know that certain problems, such as **high blood pressure** and **coronary artery disease**, begin in childhood. Doing everything possible to prevent heart disease in later life is tremendously important to parents and to everyone else who works with children. Almost all heart defects can now be successfully repaired in infancy, allowing the baby to grow into a normal adult. Once repaired, the heart needs to be kept healthy into middle and old age. The heart of each child is precious and is to be treasured.

Although the heart has been studied for many centuries, it is only in the past fifty years that scientists have come to understand how the heart develops and how particular heart problems can be recognized and treated. Today we know far more about how the heart functions and how heart problems of children can be treated than was even imagined fifty years ago. Yet the heart has more secrets to be learned.

If your child has a heart defect, you may already have learned the nature of this defect from the health care team, and you may have looked at the results of an echo test and seen the area of the heart that is involved. You may also have received a diagram of the heart and an American Heart Association booklet to take home for further study. *The Heart of a Child* will go further. It will explain how a child's heart problem can be recognized and treated, depending on the severity of the problem, and it will discuss the possible outcomes.

Much of the vocabulary used here may already be familiar to you. For example, if your child has a **ventricular septal defect** (**VSD**), you probably know that the **ventricular septum** is the wall between the two **ventricles**, which are the pumping chambers of the heart. In a ventricular septal defect that wall has not completely closed. Some ventricular septal defects are small and close by themselves; others are large and require surgery in early infancy. All of these words and concepts will be explained to you in this book. We have made every effort to explain the vocabulary used in the text, and we have included diagrams to help you visualize the textual descriptions. Terms that are defined in the Glossary appear in **boldface type** at the first mention in the text.

If you are a parent who has just learned of a defect in your child's heart, you may want to read immediately the details of that defect. The table of contents and the index will help you find the relevant passages. Later, after your child is restored to health—and most children with heart defects are—you may want to read more about how your child's heart has developed and about recent advances in treatments and research. But first, like Andrew's parents, you will begin with your own child's problem.

Andrew W. was born after a normal pregnancy; he weighed six pounds and did well in the nursery, but on the day he was scheduled to go home one of the doctors heard a heart murmur. He told Mr. and Mrs. W. that the murmur would very likely disappear. He did not think any extra tests were needed, and he alerted the pediatrician that there was a murmur. The murmur persisted, and at 3 weeks Andrew came back to the hospital for some heart tests. His parents were told that Andrew had a large ventricular septal defect. He would need to be on heart medications for a few weeks and would eventually be admitted to the hospital for heart surgery. Now, after surgery, Andrew is a lively and happy 3-year-old who acts like a normal boy in every way.

Andrew's story is repeated in many heart centers around the world every day. Yet before the defect is treated, parents will feel grief and shock at learning that their child has a heart problem. Many parents will feel a special agony because they will have to make a life-and-death decision for a newborn infant who is helpless and unable to help them decide what to do. Some will wonder anxiously if this new and precious life will end suddenly, before they have experienced the full joys of parenthood.

Only fifty years ago there was no heart surgery at all for babies like Andrew. Doctors could often tell by listening to the chest that a baby like Andrew had a ventricular defect, but they could not tell how big it was or whether additional defects were present. They could not treat it; they could only hope that the defect would get smaller on its own, that the baby would somehow grow out of it. Tests like the echocardiogram, which now provide clear pictures of the inside of the beating heart, were still far in the future.

Today is an exciting and hopeful time for most babies with heart defects, because nearly all such problems can be recognized early in life and because a wide range of treatments are available. Surgery is now possible inside the heart; it is quick and frequently effective. Some heart problems do remain difficult to treat successfully, particularly when the left ventricle, the main pumping chamber, is too small; and of course, parents of children who have multiple handicaps, both inside and outside the heart, will face particularly hard decisions. But fortunately, for about nine out of ten babies with heart problems, either the problem or defect is too mild to need any treatment at all or treatment will be successful and the child will grow to be strong and healthy.

The Heart Problems of Children

Many people think of heart problems as part of aging, a worry and concern only for middle-aged and elderly people. The **incidence** of **heart attacks** and other consequences of **atherosclerosis** and high blood pressure does, in fact, increase steadily from about 35 years of age. Heart attacks almost never happen in children. Yet some types of heart disease can occur in very young infants and even, occasionally, before birth.

About eight of every one thousand children are born with **congenital heart defects**, many of them mild and requiring no treatment. "Congenital" literally means "with birth," or dating from birth, but in fact, these defects develop early in the growth of the embryo in the womb. Approximately twenty-five thousand children are born with heart defects every year in the United States, and about five hundred forty thousand Americans who are alive today were born with such defects.

There are at least thirty-five different types of congenital heart defects. A child may be born, for example, with a defect in the walls or the valves or in the placement of the heart itself. More rarely, a child is born with a normal heart but later develops or acquires a heart problem. The heart may be damaged by an infection, usually because a virus has inflamed the heart muscle, causing **viral myocarditis**. Or a viral or bacterial infection of the thin membrane surrounding the heart may lead to **pericarditis**. Occasionally, bacteria invade the inner lining of the heart and damage the heart valves, causing **bacterial endocarditis**, which is more likely to occur in children with heart defects. Or the muscular heart wall, the **myocardium**, loses its normal strength and its powerful pump-like action after a viral infection or as part of a generalized disease, and the child develops **cardiomyopathy**, a persistent illness or weakness of the heart muscle.

Other important heart problems in children include **rheumatic heart disease** and **Kawasaki** syndrome. Although rheumatic fever has become rare in the Western world, it remains a major disease in developing countries. Kawasaki syndrome, a newly recognized disorder of very young children, occasionally leads to inflammation of the **coronary arteries**.

Abnormalities of the rate and rhythm of the heart—**arrhythmias**—can occur in children of any age. Arrhythmias vary from a mild occasional extra heartbeat that causes a sudden "thump" in the chest to severe attacks of rapid heart rate that require urgent treatment. Although many children have occasional extra heartbeats, serious abnormalities of heart rhythm are much rarer in children than in adults, and fewer than one child in one thousand needs treatment for a rhythm problem.

Mitral valve prolapse is unusual in children under the age of ten, but by the late teens it may be found in as many as thirty children in one thousand. More often than not, mitral valve prolapse is a variant of normal functioning, and it only occasionally needs any treatment. Innocent heart murmurs are heard at some time in almost half of all normal children, but these heart murmurs are not to be thought of as a problem.

How many children have heart problems?

- About eight in every one thousand children—about twenty-five thousand infants per year in this country—will be born with a heart defect. An additional forty thousand children are identified as having heart problems at the age of 1 year or older, but many of these defects are mild and require little or no treatment. Children with conditions such as Marfan's syndrome and bicuspid **aortic valve** are included in these figures.
- During childhood, about two children in one thousand will develop or acquire a new problem that affects the heart muscle or that causes serious disturbance of the heart rate or rhythm.
- Viral infections severe enough to cause symptoms, rheumatic heart disease, cardiomyopathy, and similar problems affect fewer than one in one thousand children. Malnutrition may also damage the heart, but this is unusual in the West.
- Innocent heart murmurs are heard in one of two normal children. These are not a sign of heart disease. Other murmurs can signal a defect that requires treatment.
- By the late teens perhaps thirty children per one thousand will have mitral valve prolapse, which causes many childhood heart murmurs. Very few of these, fewer than one per one thousand, will require any treatment.
- If the incidence of heart disease in adults continues at the present rate, about forty in one thousand boys and twenty in one thousand girls will have coronary artery disease, and two hundred in one thousand boys and girls will have **hypertension** (high blood pressure), by the age of 55.

Advances in Diagnosis and Treatment

Although some childhood heart problems could be recognized at the beginning of this century, no treatment was available, partly because there was little understanding of the real nature of the problems. None of the tests we now use to find out how well a child's heart is functioning had been developed. Although a good deal was known of the anatomy of defects, knowledge of anatomy is not enough. If we are to understand a defect's effects on life and health, it is vital that we know how the defect influences the function of the child's heart. Only then can we begin to envision effective treatment. Obviously, accurate diagnosis is necessary, for different types of defects need different treatments. But advances in diagnosis and in treatment influence each other. Once a treatment became available for **blue babies** (children with **cyanosis**), after Drs. Alfred Blalock and Helen Taussig performed the first successful blue baby operation in 1944, a powerful stimulus had been provided to improve diagnosis of heart defects. The dynamic of interaction goes like this:

> *Phase 1.* Some understanding, no treatment.
>
> *Phase 2.* New tests, more understanding.
>
> *Phase 3.* Treatment available—more children come for study—more understanding—effects of treatment studied—more effective treatment.

Before the 1940s, many children with heart problems died. We could not save them. Until then the diagnosis of a heart defect was an intellectual challenge only; after 1944 it was more than an intellectual challenge, because a child with a heart defect might be restored to health. Thousands of adults are alive today only because of the advances in diagnosis and treatment of heart disease made over the past fifty years.

With all these advances in treatment came an important advance in knowledge: the realization that some defects are so mild they do not need treatment. In the 1940s and 1950s physicians argued over why fewer ventricular septal defects were observed in adults than in children. Had many children with such defects died? Did the adults simply not want to see cardiologists anymore? Had some of the defects closed on their own? In 1960 Drs. John Evans and John Keith of Toronto showed conclusively that some ventricular septal defects did close without treatment. After a number of years and many studies it was agreed that children with small ventricular septal defects can lead entirely normal lives. If the defect is going to close, as it does in about one in three or four of all infants with small defects, closure usually occurs before the child is 2 years old, although closures occasionally occur even in adults. But even if closure does not occur, a small defect can be left alone. The only special precaution is the need for medication to prevent endocarditis (see chapter 14).

Certain other mild defects also require no treatment. For several years after heart surgery became possible, some families lived with great anxiety, convinced that even if their babies did not need surgery in infancy they might need it at some later time. Nowadays a long-term plan can be developed with the family and the **health team** in the child's early infancy. Families can live with more confidence about what will happen in the future.

The Growing Knowledge of the Heart

The history of the growth in knowledge of the heartbeat and the circulation of blood is a fascinating topic. André Cournand, who was one of the great pioneers of **cardiology** in this century and who won a Nobel Prize for his work on **cardiac catheterization**, has outlined this history. He says that the idea that air and blood meet within the lungs and that from this meeting blood gains a "vital essence" dates back to the Greek island of Ionia in the sixth century B.C. It took many centuries and much argument before it was known that this vital essence was oxygen, and before the circulation of the blood to and from the heart was understood. William Harvey, whose famous treatise on the heart and circulation was published in London in 1628, is generally given credit for explaining the flow of blood from the **veins** to the right ventricle to the **pulmonary artery** and lungs. Controversy continues over which others made significant early contributions.

Archaeologists have recently shown that the ancient Egyptians had detailed knowledge of many parts of the **circulatory system**. Still, for many centuries the belief persisted that blood passed from the right ventricle to the left through invisible pores in the wall or **septum** between the two ventricles, an idea that originated with the anatomist Galen in Pergamon in Asia Minor in the second century B.C. Galen made many remarkable advances in the teaching of anatomy and surgery; his influence was so strong that even when his ideas were wrong (as with the invisible pores), they survived for many centuries.

Once the circulation of the blood to and from the heart was understood, it remained for chemists to identify the gases exchanged in the lungs. In the nineteenth century Antoine Lavoisier in France and James Priestley in England demonstrated that oxygen was taken up from the air by the lungs and carbon dioxide was removed. Only in this century, with the development of heart catheterization and techniques for measuring oxygen levels in the tissues (pulse **oximetry**), has it become possible to measure exactly how much oxygen is used by an individual at different times.

Understanding of the movement of blood in the lungs and the tissues became possible after the development of the microscope. In 1661, Marcello Malpighi in Pisa first observed the flow of blood in the small vessels or **capillaries** of the lung. New knowledge is being gained even now about the intricate relationship between the heart and lungs in healthy people and, particularly, about changes in the newborn.

Blood pressure was first measured, in an ingenious way, by Stephen Hales in 1733; he put a tube, or cannula, into the **artery** of a horse, and measured the height to which blood rose in the tube. Nearly a century later, in France, Jean Leonard Poiseuille invented the mercury manometer for measuring **blood pressure** in humans. Considering how long scientists have been investigating the process of circulation, it is remarkable that everything we have learned about blood pressure was discovered so recently.

In ancient times physicians interested in the human heart had to rely on feeling the pulse. A great deal was learned from doing this, and arrhythmias of the heart were recognized long before the **electrocardiogram** was developed. Some physicians, however, equated certain pulse characteristics with specific types of diseases and personalities. In Paris in 1816, Rene Laennec listened to a patient's chest with the aid of the first "stethoscope," a quire of paper rolled into a cylinder. By listening to the heart through a stethoscope, physicians came to hear the beating heart and the normal sounds of the valves opening and closing; gradually they learned to recognize extra sounds between the normal lub-dup, lub-dup of the valves. These extra sounds or "murmurs" were soft and variable in healthy children, but some types of heart disease in which the sounds were loud could be identified by the specific timing and location of the murmurs. By early in the twentieth century certain heart problems could be diagnosed accurately by listening to the heart beat. However, some very severe problems, such as coronary artery disease, did not cause any murmurs and so eluded detection.

Although coronary arteries had been beautifully depicted in Leonardo da Vinci's drawings of the heart in the fifteenth century, and although William Harvey in the seventeenth century recognized that these arteries supply oxygen and nutrition to the heart muscle, it was not until 1912 that James Herrick showed that heart attack and sudden death could result from coronary artery blockage caused by atherosclerosis.

The myocardium differs from all other muscles in the body by virtue of its regular contraction, or beating. Although scientists discovered the spiral arrangement of the heart muscle several centuries ago, only recently has it become possible to learn how the heart is supplied with energy, and exactly how the muscle fibers move during a heartbeat. Even more exciting, heart muscle cells can now be grown in tissue culture outside the body, allowing study of the genes and proteins that are involved in the heartbeat and in heart muscle growth.

In 1879, the great French cardiologist Henri Roger understood that a certain type of murmur over the heart indicated the presence of a ventricular septal defect. In 1900 a Scottish physician, Dr. G. A. Gibson, drew an excellent diagram of the murmur of a patent **ductus arteriosus**. Physicians were beginning to understand that certain defects gave rise to certain consequences, that heart defects were neither dark mysteries nor of academic interest only. It was now possible to deduce that a certain defect was present by listening to the beating heart.

But still no treatment was available. It was believed that most heart defects shortened life, but no one knew why or how they did so. The study of the natural history of heart defects began, but it was slow work, partly because there was no "gold standard" for diagnosis while the patient was alive. A Canadian pathologist at McGill University, Dr. Maude Abbott, was one of the first to believe that treatment of heart defects would one day be possible; she began to collect full details of the medical histories and the X-ray and electrocardiographic findings (when available) of patients with heart defects. In 1936 she produced her *Atlas of Congenital Cardiac Disease* based on studies in one thousand such patients. She was encouraged in her work, which seemed a lonely and unrewarding task to many, by Dr. William Osler of Johns Hopkins, a distinguished internist, and Dr. Paul Dudley White of Boston, a renowned cardiologist. Dr. Abbott's genius and the diligence of this U.S.-Canadian collaboration brought order and a systematic approach to our knowledge of heart defects.

Pioneering Diagnostic Techniques and Treatment

Important as it was that patterns of defects could now be recognized, treatment had to wait for advances in anesthesia and surgery. The story of the development of diagnosis and treatment is fascinating; at the same time, it is a little sobering to realize how recent modern treatment is. Understanding a little about how treatment methods came about can be useful in seeing how far we have come and what still needs to be learned.

In the late 1930s and early 1940s surgeons learned to open the chest safely. They could not yet operate inside the heart, because there was no **heart-lung machine**. The first **closed-heart operations** in children were to repair patent ductus arteriosus and **coarctation** (constriction) of the **aorta**, outside the heart. Dr. Robert Gross of Boston and Dr. Clarence Crafoord of Sweden were the pioneers in this advance in the ability to repair defects outside the heart. This was a thrilling new advance. Dr. Alfred Blalock was working at that time in Tennessee on methods of repairing coarctations in the laboratory. The method that he and his technical assistant, Vivien Thomas (later Dr. Vivien Thomas), developed is not the one now used for coarctation, but the work they did then helped in the later development of the blue baby operation.

After Blalock and Thomas came to Johns Hopkins in 1940, Dr. Helen Taussig, then in charge of a special clinic devoted to heart problems in children, told them of an idea of hers. She had studied children with cyanosis, whose blue color was caused by a heart defect, and had decided that their fundamental problem was obstruction of blood flow into the lungs. She had used a fluoroscope to observe the lungs of many children with tetralogy and other problems, and she was certain that if the blood flow to their lungs could be improved they could be helped. Just then Dr. Gross in Boston was winning fame for *closing* a patent ductus in an infant and teaching other surgeons how to do it. Dr. Taussig wanted Dr. Blalock to *build* a ductus! Dr. Blalock, assisted by Vivien Thomas, did indeed build an artificial ductus—a new route for extra blood to reach the lungs. They used the subclavian artery, the vessel they had been working with in Tennessee, but instead of using it to bypass coarctation, they used it to bypass the obstruction of blood flow to the lungs. This was the Blalock-Taussig operation (see figure 13.1).

When Helen Taussig was herself an infant (she was born in 1898), there was no treatment for childhood heart disease other than **digitalis**, used for signs of **heart failure**, or aspirin, used for rheumatic fever. The lives of Dr. Taussig and the baby she is holding in the photograph (opposite) span the remarkable era when treatment of children's heart defects evolved from a dream to a reality. The photograph shows the gentleness and loving skill with which Dr. Taussig approached all children, her patients, and their families.

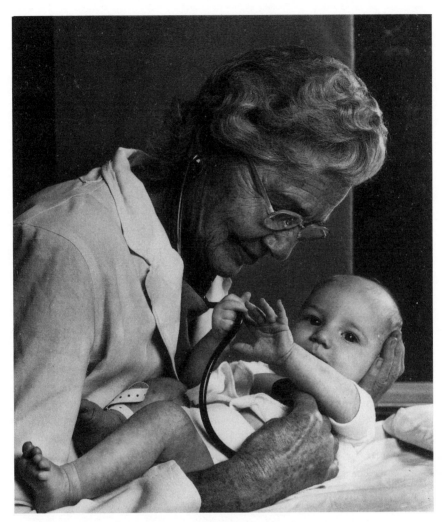

Dr. Helen Taussig in the 1980s. Photograph © Karsh.

The collaboration between Blalock and Taussig that produced the blue baby operation was an outstanding example of a brilliant idea's being taken up by someone with the skill and understanding to put it into practice. Although a child with tetralogy still had a bluer color than normal after undergoing the Blalock-Taussig operation, the obstruction of blood flow to the lungs had been bypassed.

The results were dramatic. Blue babies who previously would not have survived now did so. Those who would have survived but would have retained their intense blue color and grown into virtual invalids, irritable and unable to leave the house, could now run and play and go to school. This transformation of a few children "from blue to pink" was a medical-surgical breakthrough that swept the world and gave a tremendous impetus to efforts to learn more about the heart.

Also in the 1940s, Dr. André Cournard and his group developed the technique of cardiac catheterization. Nowadays, most of the thousands of such tests done daily around the world are performed on older people who have coronary artery disease, but in the 1940s to 1960s most cardiac catheterizations were performed on young people who had been born with heart defects. The use of catheterization findings quickly advanced the understanding of defects. We could learn more about which children with heart defects really needed treatment and which did not, even though for many who did need help no surgical technique was yet available.

It was already known, for example, that some children with ventricular septal defects had large hearts and were chronically ill, whereas others had a loud heart murmur but were otherwise healthy. Cardiac catheterization and **angiocardiography** (injection of dye into the heart, also known as angiography) led to an understanding that individual children were affected greatly by the size of the ventricular defect and the amount of flow through it. These new tests helped to clarify the physiology of defects; they made it possible to understand patterns of normal and abnormal blood flow and how they might affect the growing child. The term "flow ratios" entered the scientific lexicon. If the defect was large, a great deal of blood flowed through it from the left ventricle to the right and from the right ventricle into the lungs. As a result of excessive **pulmonary blood flow**, the lungs became congested with blood while the blood flow to the body (the **systemic blood flow**) was reduced, leading to poor growth. In the normal heart, the flow in the two circulatory systems is in perfect balance; that is, the ratio of **pulmonary** to systemic blood flow is one to one. It took some time to develop a consensus that when the blood flow from the heart to the lungs is two or more times greater than that to the body as a whole, symptoms almost always appeared.

Understanding of ventricular septal and other defects had advanced greatly by the time of the next major surgical development, the heart-lung machine. To operate safely inside the heart, surgeons needed to be able to supply blood to the brain and other vital organs during surgery. The heart-lung machine made this possible. The first successful operations to close ventricular septal defects were done in 1955 in

Minneapolis by Dr. Walton Lillehei and his team. Shortly afterward the surgeons at the Mayo Clinic in Rochester, Minnesota (at that time led by Dr. John Kirklin), started an extraordinary series of operations that helped many children. Heart-lung machines came into widespread use, and it became possible to repair the defects in **tetralogy of Fallot**. Many children with tetralogy of Fallot had a Blalock-Taussig operation first and open-heart repair later. The era of **open-heart surgery** had arrived.

Not until the 1970s was the heart-lung machine successfully used in operations on small babies. Many people worked long and hard to bring this achievement about. Sir Brian Barratt-Boyes of Auckland, New Zealand, was a leader in this phase. It was clear that the majority of deaths from heart defects occurred in infancy, but it took a long time to modify equipment to work with tiny babies. Some advances came about because surgeons by now were operating on coronary arteries and therefore needed magnifying glasses in the operating room and special small needles for sewing delicate vessels. These modifications helped greatly with the growth of successful heart surgery in young infants. Advances in specialized care of sick newborn infants, in anesthesia, and in critical-care postoperative units for children all helped make primary repair of the heart in infancy a reality. The 1980s became the era of early diagnosis; a child's heart problem could now usually be diagnosed before the child was 6 months old and, once diagnosed, could often be repaired in open-heart surgery.

Several other new developments, including new medications, had a great influence on the treatment of childhood heart problems. Effective new drugs called **diuretics** helped to treat infants and children who had excessive fluid in the lungs caused by heart failure. Other medications were produced to control abnormal heart rhythms and manipulate abnormalities of blood pressure. The advent of prostaglandin E1 treatment in the early 1980s was a major advance for sick newborns; this drug kept the ductus open in many critically ill babies while needed studies were being done and preparations were being made for surgery. Indomethacin became available to close the ductus in premature babies, thus avoiding the need for surgery altogether.

Another great advance occurred in the catheterization laboratory. Before 1966 the **cardiac** catheter was useful in diagnosis but not as a direct method of treatment. In 1966, Dr. William Rashkind of Philadelphia developed a **balloon catheter** that could enlarge a tiny opening in the **atrial septum** and help infants born with transposition of the great arteries. In 1982, Dr. Jean Kan of Johns Hopkins used a balloon

loon catheter to open up the narrowed **pulmonary valve** in children who had pulmonary **stenosis**; this method, called pulmonary **valvuloplasty**, is now used all over the world. The great breakthrough with these new methods was that surgery could now be delayed or completely avoided, and the child often could be treated without spending even one night in the hospital. Other catheters have been developed that include a device to close a patent ductus or an **atrial septal defect** (**ASD**); their future role is not yet certain.

One of the most important of all advances in heart treatment was **Doppler-echocardiography**. This is a tool of diagnosis rather than treatment, but diagnosis and treatment are, as we know, inseparable. The modern era of treatment is dependent on the speed and accuracy with which explicit motion pictures of the beating heart can be obtained. Echocardiograms began to be used in diagnosis in the 1970s, and by the mid-1980s Doppler-echocardiography was sophisticated enough to allow an accurate picture of the inside of the heart in infants and children and even in a fetus as young as 18 weeks. Although many other special tests are now available, the Doppler-echocardiogram (**echo-Doppler**) is the "gold standard" for telling us if a heart defect is present and how severe it is. Not a treatment in itself, it has helped make treatment more speedy, more precise, and more efficient.

The Principles of Modern Treatment

The overriding principle of modern treatment is to restore a child who has a heart problem to the best possible health with a minimum of tests and procedures. This principle has been made more practical by the new tool of Doppler-echocardiography. A child born with a mild defect can now lead a normal, active life. In some children a moderate heart problem can be recognized, as happened with Janine A.

> *Janine A. was an active, lively 2-year-old, although she was a little smaller than her brother Jason had been at the same age. She went to her pediatrician because of an ear infection; she had previously had a very soft heart murmur, but on the day of this visit the murmur was louder. A cardiology consultation was arranged, and Janine was found to have an atrial septal defect, a deficiency in the wall or septum between the two upper chambers of the heart. The cardiologist explained to Janine's parents that the defect could lead to enlargement of the heart and abnormal heart rhythms when*

Janine became an adult; the cardiologist recommended surgical re-pair. Although such a defect can be repaired at any age, Janine underwent surgery before she was 4, because the heart returns to normal size more readily in a young child. She did very well and has had no sign of any problem in the three years since her operation.

For a child like Janine, an early referral to a cardiologist allows a plan for treatment to be developed, so that the child can be fully active and can return for surgical closure of the defect, usually between 1 and 4 years of age. Sometimes a defect is found that becomes more severe as the child grows; for example, a child with pulmonary stenosis may not need treatment with pulmonary valvuloplasty until 4 years of age or perhaps older.

Sometimes in the past severe heart defects, such as those that cause signs of heart failure or cyanosis, were treated with medications, reviewed by many catheterization tests, and repaired in several different operations. Now, however, surgery in infancy is almost always the best course. The principle of treatment is to use medications for only a brief time—to relieve signs of congestion in the body and lungs—and then go on to surgery, a course that has completely altered the outlook for infants with large ventricular septal defects. In past years such a baby would remain on medications for months, perhaps years, growing poorly and often requiring hospital admission several times a year because any viral illness would make the congestion in the lungs much worse. Now such a child goes to the hospital once, briefly, for surgery and then goes home not needing any medications. The parents can look forward with joy and expectation to the day when their child will go off to school, as happy and mischievous as any of the other children!

For babies born with critical heart defects, those requiring urgent treatment in the newborn period, the new treatments can be wonderful. For example, until the mid-1960s, an infant born with transposition had less than a 5-percent chance of reaching his or her first birthday. Now successful surgery can usually be done in the first week of life. The baby who before would have lived precariously and briefly, always blue and short of breath, is lively, healthy, and a normal color.

By contrast, another infant born at the same time and in an area where equally excellent cardiac care is available may be in the hospital for a month or longer and may need several operations. This difficult and stressful course is the exception, however, and is usually the consequence of a severe and **complex heart defect**. By complex we mean that there are abnormalities in several different areas of the heart, not just one; often one of the ventricles or principal chambers has failed to develop, or a major artery or heart valve is completely blocked. Early repair by one operation is usually not possible. Sometimes the defect in the heart itself is not particularly complex, and it is additional major problems outside the heart that make treatment difficult and prolonged.

The knowledge that most babies can now be successfully treated with only a brief stay in the hospital does not make it any easier for families of infants who have multiple problems. Fortunately, even after a prolonged and difficult start in life, more and more babies with complex defects eventually go home and do well.

As many infectious diseases and childhood illnesses pass into history, the presence of any defect or illness in a child becomes increasingly exceptional and thus in some ways even more difficult for the family. When families were larger and childhood illnesses were more common, young parents with an ailing child had friends and neighbors with ailing children of their own; even if the illness was transitory, there was a shared bond of understanding. Now, when most families are small and many children have no illness except for an occasional cold, the parents of a child with a heart problem, even one that is mild and easily treated, can feel isolated. A good health team can do a great deal to lift this sense of isolation. Together, the health team, the family, and the child may participate in a triangle of understanding.

The Triangle of Understanding

Medical writers often imply that families won't comply with medical instructions because they just don't understand the problem. Our own experience suggests that almost all families can and do understand the basic principles of heart problems, given a little time and appropriate diagrams and illustrations. Parents often do find it difficult to understand the many different terms used by so many different people, or why one member of the health team has emphasized a glowing, healthy future for the child while another has seemed to concentrate on risks and hazards. If the parents and the health team think of the child as the focus and realize that each member of the triangle—child,

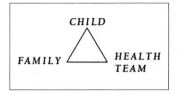

In order best to help the child with a heart problem, **the triangle of understanding** involving family, child, and health team must be strong and durable. Understanding is a three-way process. *Cor ad cor loquiter:* heart must speak to heart.

parent, and health team member—can teach the others, a loving triangle of understanding can be maintained.

The health team can learn from the parents how to watch for subtle signs that the baby is uncomfortable or is trying to ask for help. The parents can learn from the nurses skilled and gentle handling of a baby in crisis. The baby, and his or her future well-being, is the apex of the triangle and the theme of this book. We have been fortunate enough to know many pioneering patients and their families, and in this book we will share some of their experiences. Knowing such patients and their friends leaves one full of gratitude, hope, and a continuing sense of wonder at the marvels of the heart of a child.

Part I

IDENTIFYING A CHILD'S HEART PROBLEM AND ITS CAUSES

Chapter 1

Recognizing a Heart Problem

In some ways it is harder to identify a heart problem in a child than in an adult. An adult can describe shortness of breath on climbing stairs or a crushing discomfort in the chest on walking—symptoms that immediately direct a physician's attention to the heart. An infant has to wait for the family or physician to recognize that a problem exists. Some years ago, Dr. Proctor Harvey of Georgetown used a "five-finger approach" to adult heart problems that can prove helpful in recognizing and defining the problem exactly in infants as well. His approach draws together, as a guide to diagnosis, what the family can see, what the physician can see and hear, and the results of various tests.

What the Family Can See: The Child's History

Although a baby cannot say in words that he or she is short of breath, the family may notice that the baby is breathing faster than normal even when asleep. Sometimes this rapid breathing is present from birth; sometimes a baby may begin life breathing like other newborns but between 1 and 3 months of age start to breathe fast and sound as if he or she is panting after the slightest exertion. This change from a normal breathing pattern to rapid panting may be a sign that the lungs are becoming congested because of a heart defect. Or the parents may see that although the baby starts to feed eagerly, he or she soon begins to sweat and become irritable. By no means are all feeding problems in infancy the result of a heart problem, but when poor feeding is combined with rapid breathing and sweating, the baby may be trying to tell us that the exertion of feeding is tiring. Sometimes a family may notice, in addition to slow growth and feeding problems, that the baby's lips and nails are blue, a condition that is more obvious when the baby cries or feeds.

The family reports these clues, or this history, to the pediatrician, and thus the first step in diagnosis is taken. Parents may tell the pediatrician that their baby is experiencing

- Shortness of breath, especially when feeding or crying
- Tiredness and sweating during feeding
- Blueness (cyanosis) of the lips and nail beds, made more intense by crying or activity
- Slow growth, especially slowness in gaining weight

Older children may notice symptoms such as chest pains or shortness of breath after exercise or the sudden onset of palpitations, and may tell their parents or physician, but younger children can only show us the signs of trouble. The "first finger" in Dr. Harvey's approach is a family's noticing these signs of trouble and reporting them to the pediatrician.

What the Physician Can See and Hear: The Physical Examination

Alerted by the family to the possibility of a problem, the physician will check the baby's rate of breathing (Is it rapid for the child's age?) and search for any signs of heart failure, including an enlarged heart or a large liver; look for a bluish discoloration of the lips and nail beds; check for an abnormal heart rhythm or pulses; and listen for a heart murmur (an added sound over the heart's normal sound).

Although an infant or child may appear perfectly healthy, the physician may hear a murmur and recommend further studies. A heart murmur in an otherwise healthy child means either no heart trouble at all or a mild heart defect. Sometimes a murmur is caused by a small patent ductus, for which surgery is recommended. The idea that a healthy, active baby might need heart surgery is particularly difficult for parents to accept or understand, and the family and the health team (the physician, the cardiologist, and others) will review together the exact nature of the problem and options for treatment.

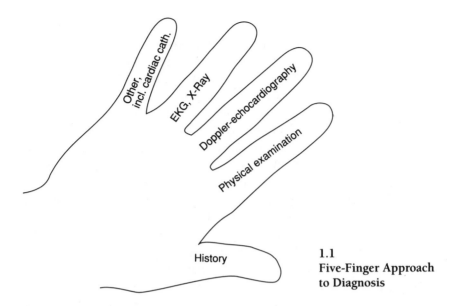

1.1
Five-Finger Approach
to Diagnosis

Because most defects of the heart walls are small and do not cause symptoms, they are usually recognized when a murmur is detected during a regularly scheduled checkup (the "second finger" in figure 1.1). The murmur may occasionally be so loud (as in a ventricular septal defect, a problem in the heart wall) that the mother will feel it with her hand while bathing or fondling her baby. This "thrill" is caused by a loud murmur that produces a vibration on the chest wall with each heartbeat. It feels almost like the purring of a cat, but the timing is different. A cat purrs when breathing; the thrill and murmur follow the timing of the heartbeat. Almost always, however, the murmur is first detected by a physician or nurse. Its quality will indicate whether a heart defect is likely or not. The timing of the physician's referral to a cardiologist will depend a great deal on how well the baby is growing and on the type of defect suspected. Sometimes the baby needs early and urgent treatment.

If the family physician or pediatrician refers the parents to a cardiologist, this specialist will confirm the history with the family and then observe the baby and the family together. Time spent in observation of the baby allows for assessment of general health and the severity of any symptoms (for example, the baby's blueness and the pattern of breathing). This quiet time even before a stethoscope is used lets parents and cardiologist become comfortable with each other, focusing together on the infant and his or her special needs. Later, a detailed examination of the heart sounds and the timing and loudness of the murmur can provide useful clues to any defect. The cardiologist will recommend special tests to identify the heart problem or to confirm what he or she has suspected from the examination.

To take one example, a baby boy may have an anxious expression, a little scowl. As he sits up in his mother's or father's arms, he breathes at twice the usual rate and looks around in an alert and worried way. The cardiologist observes that he is thin and learns that he has been growing slowly. A loud heart murmur is heard. His mother reports that he feeds eagerly but that he quickly gets tired and fussy. He sweats around the head. This baby has the look of someone whose heart is beginning to fail; it was a tragic sight before effective treatment methods had been developed, and it is still very touching.

The cardiologist is almost certain that a large defect exists in the ventricular septum of the baby's heart. The cardiologist's diagnosis will be greatly helped by the findings of an echo-Doppler test, also called a Doppler-echocardiogram, and an electrocardiogram. The exact size and position of the large defect as well as any additional defects will be seen on the echo study. With the echo-Doppler, the pressure in the pulmonary artery can be measured with a great deal of accuracy.

Diagnostic Tests

Doppler-echocardiogram

One of the first tests the cardiologist may recommend is called the Doppler-echocardiogram. It can identify many heart defects.

In fact, heart defects can sometimes be identified even before birth. Many young mothers reading this book will have had an ultrasound test during their pregnancy and will remember the excitement of seeing their baby move and watching the rapid heartbeat. Viewing the heart of the growing baby at 16 to 20 weeks, the physician can see nearly all parts of the heart clearly. If, on the ultrasound, there is a suspicion of a heart problem, more detailed views of the heart can then be obtained in a heart center, where obstetricians and cardiologists work together. In such cases, diagnosis comes before symptoms.

Certain severe heart defects can be recognized as early as 16 weeks. As more and more mothers have fetal ultrasound tests, it seems likely that even earlier diagnosis will soon be possible. Preparation can then be made for emergency treatment at birth, if necessary, and perhaps the delivery itself can even take place in a heart center. At the present time, only about 1 percent of all heart defects are detected by fetal **echocardiography**, but this proportion is likely to increase rapidly.

Although this book will emphasize heart defects, it is vital to remember that most **fetal Doppler-echocardiography** is used to help us know more about the normal heart and how it grows. It will be reassuring to parents who have already had a baby with a heart defect to know early in a pregnancy that the new baby's heart has four normal-sized chambers and is beating as it should.

The Doppler-echocardiogram has been very helpful in understanding childhood heart problems. It has been particularly helpful for critically ill newborns, by quickly defining the nature and severity of any heart defect that developed in the womb. It has made planning further tests and surgery much faster and more accurate than in the past. In older children with heart murmurs or other symptoms, this test can help define clearly whether a heart problem does indeed exist.

Doppler-echocardiography (the "third finger" in figure 1.1) is such an extraordinary advance that its full impact is not yet realized. In Galen's time the heart could be felt only through the chest wall; by the nineteenth century, it could be examined with a stethoscope. But now, the beating heart can be seen, the thickness of the muscle in the heart wall can be measured, and the valves of the heart can be observed as they open and close. Several different views of the heart can be obtained (figures 1.2 and 1.3). Some views are particularly useful in showing the ventricles or pumping chambers. Other views can show the size and relationship of the aorta and pulmonary artery, the vessels carrying blood from the heart to the body and lungs. If any obstruction exists in the child's heart, the severity of that obstruction can be measured.

During the test the child lies on a bed or examining table. The technician or doctor holds a small device, known as a transducer, on the chest wall. Mothers who have had an abdominal ultrasound test during pregnancy can explain to a child old enough to understand how this will feel and why it is important to keep still during the thirty to forty-five minutes the test usually takes. It is not painful, although the child may feel a vibration on the chest wall; occasionally a young child will need sedating. Many older children enjoy watching the television image of their own beating heart; some take home a print of the picture to show friends or schoolmates.

The echocardiograph uses high-frequency ultrasound waves transmitted into the body; echoes returning from the surfaces of the heart and other structures are electronically plotted and recorded. The same principle is used by the bat when it "sees in the dark," as described by Randall Jarrell.

> All night, in happiness, she hunts and flies.
> Her high sharp cries
> Like shining needlepoints of sound
> Go out into the night and, echoing back,
> Tell her what they have touched.
> She hears how far it is, how big it is,
> Which way it's going:
> She lives by hearing.
>
> —Randall Jarrell, *Bats*

The echocardiogram and Doppler tests are done at the same time. Both use ultrasound waves to study the heart. The echo is used primarily to look at the anatomy of the various chambers and arteries, and in measurements of chamber size and heart function. The Doppler study is used to measure the speed with which waves travel and to measure pressure changes across the heart valves. Doppler color flow mapping superimposes color on the image received back from the heart: this color mapping is helpful in showing the direction of flow across valves, or through small defects which might otherwise be difficult to detect.

The Doppler test analyzes the same ultrasound waves the echocardiogram records, but it obtains additional information. The Doppler-echo uses the ultrasound signals back-scattered by moving bodies, primarily red blood cells moving through the heart. It also analyzes the returning signal for changes in the frequency of the sound waves (the **Doppler shift**), which help determine how fast the blood is moving in different areas and the velocity of blood flow and, therefore, what changes in pressure occur across heart valves caused by thickening or obstruction.

Taping the sound of blood flowing through your child's heart allows you not only to hear the beating heart but also to see it, as in the echocardiogram. This is because ultrasound waves sent into the chest are reflected back from the heart and displayed on a television screen, with the images sent back from the solid structures of the heart recorded on videotape. This technique makes it possible to see all four chambers of the heart, to measure the size of the aorta and pulmonary

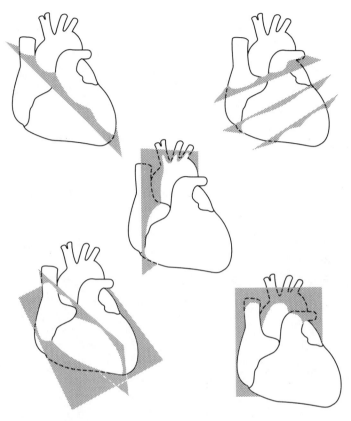

1.2. Common Echocardiographic Views. The view shown *top left*, the *long axis view*, is used to show the left ventricle, the aorta, and the mitral valve. The *short axis view*, seen in the lower slice *top right*, is useful for measuring the size and function of the left ventricle. Other views shown may be used to obtain a complete picture of the child's heart.

artery, and to determine whether the wall of the ventricle is thicker than normal. The way the ventricle contracts and the volume of blood the ventricle pushes out with each beat can be measured. Measuring the ratio of the cavity size during contraction to the size at rest provides an excellent clue to the functioning of the heart muscle.

With a Doppler probe the speed or velocity of the blood flow across heart valves and other openings can be measured, making it possible to estimate the pressures in the heart and to check the severity of any obstruction or blockage. The sound of blood flow through the heart may be heard by those in the room and can be recorded on videotape.

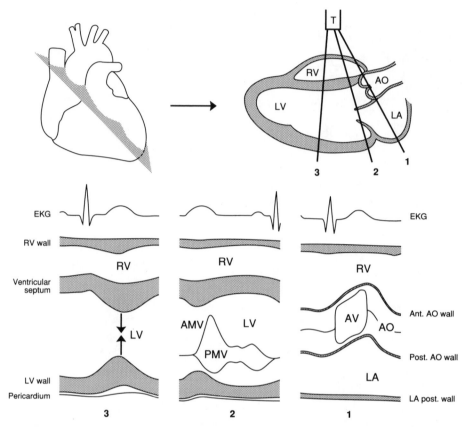

1.3. Long Axis Echocardiographic View. With the transducer (*T*) angled in different ways on the chest, different views of the heart can be recorded. In view 1 the aorta (*AO*), aortic valve (*AV*), and left atrium (*LA*) are seen; in view 2 the right ventricle (*RV*) and left ventricle (*LV*) and the two leaflets of the mitral valve (*MV*) are seen opening and closing: *AMV* is the anterior and *PMV* the posterior mitral valve leaflet; in view 3 the size of the left ventricle and the thickness of its wall can be measured. Also, the movement of the left ventricle can be seen and an accurate measurement obtained of how well it is functioning. Adapted from Harvey Feigenbaum, "Clinical Applications of Echocardiography," *Progress in Cardiovascular Diseases* 14 (May 1972): 531–559.

Usually, families find reviewing the videotape of the echocardiogram extremely helpful. The sight of the heart beating so actively is reassuring. The two-dimensional views and clear images seem more real and are more understandable than X-rays or drawings: it is also helpful for parents to receive a heart diagram to take home for review and discussion.

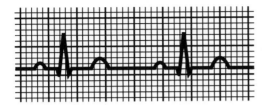

1.4.
Normal Electrocardiogram.
Here, one lead from a child's
EKG shows a normal heart
rate and rhythm.

Electrocardiogram

Another test the cardiologist may feel necessary is an electrocardiogram or EKG (the "fourth finger" in figure 1.1) Electrocardiography has allowed us to understand the normal and abnormal rhythms of the heart and the normal variations in heart rate with age.

The EKG is particularly useful in detecting abnormal heart rates or rhythms. Figure 1.4, for example, shows two heartbeats from a child with a normal rate and rhythm. An EKG can show the exact nature of any rhythm abnormality and help determine whether treatment has been effective. When a heart murmur is heard or a child has symptoms suggesting a heart problem, an EKG will be ordered as a screening test. It is used to detect heart problems such as signs of overwork or **ventricular hypertrophy** or damage to heart muscle caused by a heart attack or a toxin.

What specific information does the EKG provide about the child's heart? The EKG records each heartbeat, the electrical impulse or wave that travels through the heart. Electrodes placed on the child's chest measure this electrical activity and record it. Twelve different leads are usually recorded so that the passage of the electrical impulse through the heart chambers can be followed and compared with the passage expected in a normal child of the same age. If the EKG is found to be completely normal, a severe heart problem is unlikely.

Although electrocardiography is less important in diagnosing heart problems in children than in adults, it is very valuable nonetheless as a screening test in children when there is any suspicion of a heart problem or as part of a follow-up cardiac evaluation. It does not show the same detailed anatomy and function of the heart that Doppler-echocardiography provides, but it is helpful in many children.

Other Studies

As anyone who has watched medical programs on TV knows, there seem to be an infinite number of possible medical tests. We mention here only those frequently recommended to clarify children's heart problems (the "fifth finger" in figure 1.1). These include X-rays and fluoroscopy, cardiac catheterization, **exercise testing, Holter monitoring**, tilt-table testing, and blood tests and oximetry. Nuclear scanning tests are used in a few children if other studies have not resolved some difficult questions about the flow of blood to the heart muscle or to the lungs. Other more rarely used tests, such as **magnetic resonance imaging (MRI), computerized axial tomography (CAT) scanning**, and **electrophysiologic studies (EPS)**, are described briefly in the Glossary.

X-ray of the chest and fluoroscopy

In the past, X-rays and fluoroscopy (looking at the chest through an X-ray screen) were used a great deal to identify heart disease. Since the echo-Doppler has become so widely used, many pediatric heart centers now use X-rays only occasionally, and fluoroscopy not at all, in most cases of suspected childhood heart problems.

A chest X-ray will show an enlargement of the heart or an abnormal flow of blood to the lungs. Although certain X-ray patterns of heart shape and size are "typical" of certain heart defects and X-rays therefore have a certain value, chest X-rays, as noted, are usually not ordered now. Echo-Doppler studies have replaced them. A chest X-ray is almost always done when a child faces heart surgery, however, to make certain that there is no lung infection that could make anesthesia riskier.

Cardiac catheterization and cineangiocardiography

Cardiac catheterization or **cineangiocardiography** has been widely used for diagnosis since the 1940s and, more recently, for treatment. In this test a thin, hollow tube (catheter) is passed from the vein in the groin up into the heart where it measures oxygen levels and pressures in the different chambers.

Although now used only in patients with heart problems, cardiac catheterization has clearly defined the normal pressures in the different chambers and the oxygen used by the body. It has also determined the output of the heart, that is, the amount of blood pumped out with each heartbeat for people of different ages and with different types of heart problems.

This is an **invasive** test, that is, it enters the body. It can be done under local anesthesia and sedative drugs so that a general anesthetic is not needed. The test is done in a laboratory that specializes in such childhood studies. Most children do not need to come into the hospital overnight, but instead can stay with their parents in a nearby Same Day Care Center before and after the test. A Same Day or Ambulatory Care Center may be at the hospital, or it may be located in a separate building. In either case, children can stay in a room with their parents until the catheterization test, and then come back to the same room for two or three hours before going home. If a child has any discomfort or feels nauseous after the test, a nurse is at hand, but the problems of staying away from home overnight are avoided. Most children's heart centers supply excellent booklets to help the family and the child know exactly what will be done. Some use dolls and puppets to prepare preschool children for such a test.

Once the catheter has been passed up from the vein in the groin to the heart, small samples of blood can be withdrawn from each heart chamber. The amount of oxygen in the blood in each chamber will be measured. (Figure 1.5 shows that normally the oxygen level is the same on the right side of the heart—in the right **atrium**, the right ventricle, and the pulmonary artery.)

A device inside the catheter called a pressure transducer measures pressure in the various heart chambers. By analyzing the pressure readings and the oxygen levels in the heart chambers, the medical staff can tell if there is an obstruction of one of the heart valves or a defect in the septum or wall between the chambers.

After blood studies and pressure measurements are completed, a contrast material dye is injected into the heart to highlight any existing defect; this dye shows up as an intense white on the X-ray film. Special X-ray pictures called **cineangiograms** can be reviewed together by the cardiologist and the family after the test is completed and when the child is comfortably back in bed in the Same Day Care Center. The dye is rapidly removed from the bloodstream by the kidneys and does not linger in the body.

In earlier years, cardiac catheterization was required for many children, but because the echo-Doppler tests are now so accurate and so widely available, cardiac catheterization is seldom done except shortly before heart surgery, particularly when the child's heart has more than one defect. Cardiac catheterization can add information not available from other tests, such as the pressure in different heart chambers, and anatomical details of the arteries to the lungs and vessels outside the heart. A good picture of the small arteries in the lungs can be obtained, and sometimes additional defects not detected by echocardiography can be identified. In the past, cardiac catheterization was the most ac-

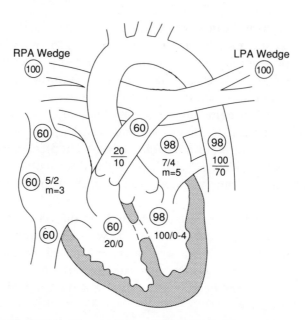

1.5. Cardiac Catheterization. *Oxygen saturations* in this normal heart diagram are shown in circles: for example, the blood in the left heart chambers is almost fully saturated (98 to 100 percent) with oxygen. The saturations in the right side of the heart are lower and do not normally vary between the right atrium and pulmonary artery (a rise in saturation in the right ventricle may mean a ventricular septal defect is present, and that fully oxygenated blood is coming from left to right through the defect). *Pressure readings* are shown in the aorta (100/70) and the different heart chambers. The pressure level in the right ventricle and pulmonary artery is usually only about one-fifth that in the left ventricle and aorta. The pressures in the heart vary with age and with the type of heart problem. Key: *RPA* = right pulmonary artery; *LPA* = left pulmonary artery.

curate way of detecting an abnormal course of one of the coronary arteries, a course that might make surgical repair (e.g., for tetralogy) more difficult; the echo-Doppler now answers this particular question almost as accurately, but it does not illustrate the small lung arteries quite as well as cardiac catheterization. It is likely that as echo-Doppler studies become increasingly sophisticated, fewer cardiac catheterizations will be performed. Thus, the role of the cardiac catheter in diagnosis and treatment is still evolving. Eventually fewer and fewer children will need catheter tests for simple defects clearly detected by echocardiography, and the catheterization laboratory will be used mainly for complex problems and for certain treatments.

In some children a cardiac catheter is used for both diagnosis and treatment. In these children a special balloon catheter is inserted into the heart to dilate a narrowed valve, as is done in most cases of pulmonary valve stenosis. Catheter balloon valvuloplasty, as it is called, is a remarkable advance that permits many children to avoid surgery altogether.

Catheters can be used in cardiac biopsy to obtain a small sample of heart muscle in children with diseases of the myocardium (see chapter 8). They can also be used before and after a heart transplant. Biopsy is done only in a small subgroup of children who need catheter studies. Some risks are associated with catheterization, particularly when it is performed on a small, sick infant. The cardiologist can help parents assess these risks and compare them to the benefit of the procedure for their child.

Occasionally, a child with a severe rhythm disorder of the heart will require an electrophysiologic study, a complex test in which catheters map the course of the electrical impulse inside the heart chambers. This type of test should be done only in a center that has made a special study of severe arrhythmias in children (see chapter 8).

Exercise testing

Exercise testing is used to see whether a child can safely exert himself or herself to a level other children of that age reach without showing abnormal heart rhythms or any EKG sign of an inadequate supply of oxygen to the heart. The test is used most often in children who have arrhythmias or abnormalities of heart muscle. Children aged 7 and older can exercise on a treadmill; younger children can use a stationary bicycle. In both methods, a system of graded exercise is used: the child starts slowly and gradually increases the exercise while an EKG tracing is continuously recorded. Blood pressure is checked regularly during the test, and in some laboratories the amount of oxygen used during exercise is also measured. By comparing the level of exercise achieved with normal tables for children of the same height and weight, a physician can assess the level of a child's fitness. Even more important, the test can show whether an existing abnormal rhythm becomes worse after exercise and thus needs treatment.

Exercise testing is beginning to be widely used in children who have both heart and lung disease. It can be valuable in clarifying whether a child who still tires easily after heart surgery does so because of lack of conditioning or because there is still a problem in the way the heart and lungs respond to exercise. Such tests are also increasingly used for teenagers with symptoms of chest pain and shortness of breath—symptoms that may or may not be related to the heart.

Holter monitoring

A child, like an adult, may complain of palpitations or an irregular heartbeat, although an EKG taken at rest is normal. It may then be useful to record an EKG continuously for twenty-four to forty-eight hours on a tape recorder, while the child is at home, both active and asleep. This record (Holter monitoring) can then be analyzed to detect any abnormal heartbeats and determine whether medication is needed.

Monitoring is also useful, even in the absence of symptoms, after heart operations that sometimes cause arrhythmia. Also, children who are on medication for arrhythmias may be monitored to follow the success of treatment. Despite its inconvenience, a Holter, in addition, can be useful in identifying palpitations that are not a problem (benign) and in managing persistent arrhythmias. Because the tape recorder for the EKG is a little bulky, some children feel self-conscious about wearing it unless they can persuade their friends, as some do, that it is a new kind of camera case or portable tape player.

In some arrhythmias that occur only occasionally, other kinds of event monitors can be turned on when the child or observer notes something abnormal, and a recording can be made of exactly what the heart rhythm was during the display of symptoms.

Tilt-table testing

If a child or teenager has fainting spells (syncope), blood pressure and pulse rate may be checked while the child is lying flat and then again upright on a "tilt table." This test is useful in planning future treatment to avoid more such episodes.

Blood tests and pulse oximetry

Additional tests may be requested for blue or cyanotic infants and children. Tests to measure the level of hemoglobin in the blood may be recommended, for example, to help decide on the best timing for surgery, or a pulse oximeter may be placed on the child's finger to measure the oxygen level in the blood both at rest and during activity.

Blood tests useful in tetralogy, for example, include measuring the level of hemoglobin and hematocrit with a tiny quantity of blood obtained from a finger. When the oxygen level in the blood is lower than normal, a complex chain of events may lead to a rise in hemoglobin, as the body seeks to compensate for too little oxygen, resulting in a kind of "overshoot," with too many red blood cells and too much hemoglobin. If the level is much higher than the usual 40 percent, the blood is thicker and stickier than normal, increasing the chance of blood **clots** and stroke. Some babies with tetralogy (see chapter 5) or other cyanotic heart defects have a bad combination of too many red blood cells, each containing too little hemoglobin—a particular risk in babies who have had any recent infection or who are feeding poorly. Iron medication for anemia may be needed.

Oximetry is a way of measuring the oxygen level in the blood when the child is both awake and asleep. It is particularly useful when blueness or cyanosis is mild when the child is at rest, because it can show conclusively whether the level of oxygen in the arteries falls with exertion or not. A pulse oximeter on the finger does not disturb the baby.

Do all children need heart tests?

Must every child be checked for heart problems? The answer is a resounding NO!

Most children never need any of these tests. A healthy, active child who is growing normally and is free of heart murmurs can happily avoid all the modern technology outlined in this chapter. Indeed, a recent study has shown that pediatricians are usually extremely successful at concluding from the history and examination of a child whether he or she has a heart problem. But when heart disease is known to be present or strongly suspected, any of these tests may prove useful and often the results are reassuring.

Chapter 2

The Developing Heart

The heart of a child is a constant source of wonder and delight. Today we know more about the human heart than ever before, yet this knowledge cannot lessen our joy in watching a healthy child at play or change our sense of awe at the complexities of the heart.

The human heart is not a simple pump, as some have described it. The heart of a child is a remarkable, complex living structure that beats continuously and rhythmically, responding with speed and sensitivity to the growing child's needs. With each beat it sends blood that contains oxygen and nutrients to all parts of the body. It beats inside one of the world's great wonders, another remarkable complex living structure, the growing child.

Parents who fear that their child may have a heart problem, or who have just learned of a defect in their child's heart, will want to know how the heart develops normally and what can go wrong in this development and why.

How the Heart Works: The Heartbeat, the Heart Rate, and the Blood Flow

The heart (figures 2.1 and 2.2) is a muscular four-chambered organ that lies under the sternum, or breastbone. It is usually easy to feel the apex or tip of the heart in the left side of the chest, just below the nipple. In young children, because the chest wall is thin, you can often see the heart beating. If you feel your own pulse or heartbeat while you are

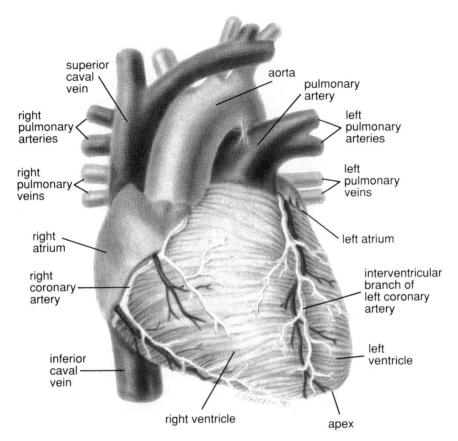

superior caval vein

aorta

pulmonary artery

right pulmonary arteries

left pulmonary arteries

right pulmonary veins

left pulmonary veins

right atrium

left atrium

right coronary artery

interventricular branch of left coronary artery

inferior caval vein

left ventricle

right ventricle

apex

2.1. The Human Heart

sitting relaxed, you will find that the rate is somewhere between fifty and eighty beats per minute. The beats follow one another regularly, although if you take a deep breath the rate speeds up a little as you breathe in and slows as you breathe out. The rate of the heart varies with age and with the demands of the body. A baby's heart rate is likely to be faster than an adult's, probably around 100 beats per minute. A young baby's heart rate will also vary more than an adult's, and changes in rate will occur more quickly.

Heart rhythm is regular, but not metronomically so. With each heartbeat, both the left and right ventricles contract (figure 2.3). During the time of ventricular contraction, known as **systole**, the right ventricle pumps blood into the pulmonary artery to reach the lungs. Simultaneously, the left ventricle pumps blood out through the open aortic valve to reach the body. When you feel the heartbeat in your own

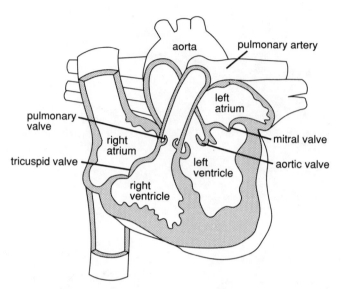

2.2. The Normal Heart. The normal heart is separated into right and left sides by walls (septa); each heart chamber has a wall around it consisting of a delicate membrane, the *pericardium* (not labeled); a layer of muscle, the *myocardium* (*shown shaded*); and a smooth inner lining, the *endocardium* (not labeled).

The normal heart has four valves, the tricuspid and pulmonary valves on the right, the mitral and aortic valves on the left. The coronary arteries are omitted here, but are shown in figure 2.1. All defects and diseases of the heart affect one or more of the structures shown in these two figures.

chest, you are feeling this pumping motion of the left ventricle. When you feel your pulse, you are feeling the blood pulsing in your radial artery, the artery in your wrist; the ventricle has contracted, sending blood into the aorta and from there to the radial artery. Ventricular systole has occurred again.

Between one heartbeat and the next, the ventricles relax. Blood flows from the veins into the right atrium; at the same time, the left atrium receives blood returning from the lungs through the pulmonary veins (figure 2.4). The time in the cardiac cycle when blood is returning to the heart, the time of ventricular relaxation, is known as **diastole**. As the **atria** contract, the valves between the atria and ventricles open, allowing blood to pass into the ventricles. As the next ventricular contraction or systole begins, the pulmonary valve and the aortic valve open and the cycle of the beating heart begins again.

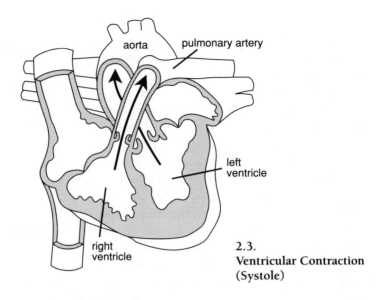

2.3.
**Ventricular Contraction
(Systole)**

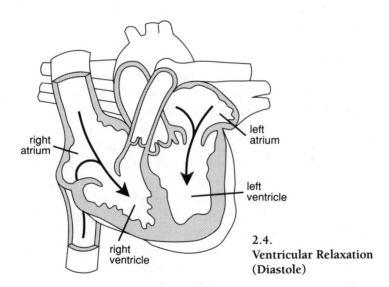

2.4.
**Ventricular Relaxation
(Diastole)**

From the arteries, blood passes into tiny vessels called capillaries; in these vessels the vital exchange of oxygen and chemicals needed by the body tissues takes place. In the lung capillaries, a new supply of oxygen is absorbed and carbon dioxide is given up. From the capillaries, blood passes back to the veins to reach the heart for a new heart cycle.

Each of the four chambers and four valves of the heart is important. If an atrium or ventricle fails to grow normally during gestation it will be too small, or perhaps absent altogether, and the heart will not be able to function properly after birth. The heart valves need to be normally formed so that they can open and close efficiently with each heartbeat. The normal pulmonary and aortic valves each have three strong yet delicate cusps or leaflets. (Figure 2.2, the diagram of the normal heart, shows only two leaflets because the drawing is not in three dimensions.) The number of leaflets in each valve—including the three in the tricuspid and two in the mitral valve—and their shape and structure have been demonstrated to be remarkably efficient mechanically. Perhaps we should not be surprised to learn this. Even while you are sitting quietly reading this book, your own aortic valve is being forced open seventy or more times per minute by blood leaving the left ventricle at the high pressure of over 100 mm Hg (millimeters of mercury). Less than 1 second later the valve closes again, without any leakage, at a pressure of 70 to 85 mm Hg. You can calculate how often your valve has already done this by calculating the minutes in a day and the days in your life so far.

But if a heart valve has thickened or narrowed, normal blood flow will be obstructed or delayed. A narrowed valve increases the pressure within the chambers, thus making the heart work harder. If a valve is "floppy" or has inadequate leaflets, it will not close properly and will allow blood to leak backward. Leaking, or "insufficiency," of a valve can greatly increase the work the heart needs to perform.

For normal circulation, the arteries and veins also need to be healthy and free of clots or blockage. In particular, normal coronary arteries are essential, because they supply oxygen and nutrition to all parts of the heart. In addition, the myocardium, or heart muscle, needs to be healthy. Each heart-muscle cell contains fibers made up of chains of proteins called actin and myosin. Tiny structures inside each fiber, called mitochondria, supply the energy necessary for the actin and myosin chains to slide over one another at each contraction of muscle that forces blood from the heart.

The rate and rhythm of the normal heart are controlled by messages sent from the brain through specialized nerve fibers to the conducting system of the heart. Messages from the nerves act like electrical impulses, causing the myocardium to start the contraction process.

After birth, the body's two circulatory systems, pulmonary and systemic, are separated from each other by walls called septa. The right atrium is separated from the left by a thin wall, the atrial septum; the right ventricle is separated from the left by a thicker muscular wall, the ventricular septum.

In the pulmonary circulation blood is carried to the lungs to obtain a fresh supply of oxygen; in the systemic circulation this new supply of oxygen is carried to the body. In this book, as in others, the term "blue" is used to describe blood returning from the veins to the pulmonary circulation, and the term "red" to describe the arterial blood. In reality, any blood lost looks red; arterial blood is a brighter red because it contains more oxygen. Venous ("blue") blood is closer to purple.

The heart and lungs depend on each other; the health of each affects the other. If the heart muscle weakens, fluid backs up in the lungs, which become congested; if the lungs are severely diseased, as in cystic fibrosis, too little oxygen is taken up at each heartbeat and eventually all parts of the body suffer from lack of oxygen.

The normal heart of a healthy child still holds many mysteries. The new science of molecular biology is beginning to reveal some of the interactions of heart cells underlying the rhythmicity and responsiveness of the normal heart.

How the Heart Develops in the Embryo and Fetus

All defects in the heart and all types of heart disease are caused by some disturbance in the development or functioning of one of the parts of the normal heart. The heart begins as a simple, almost primitive structure, quite different from the complex four-chambered organ that is the center of a child's circulation. It begins with two tubes that appear side by side in the midline of the embryo; these tubes join or fuse together and produce the early heart tube. This cardiac tube, made of muscle cells only about three to five cell layers thick, becomes the cardiac muscle or myocardium. The myocardial (heart muscle) cells surround a collection of complex proteins called **cardiac jelly**, which later plays a big role in forming the heart valves. The cardiac tube is lined with a delicate single layer of cells that will later become the inner lining of the heart, or **endocardium**.

By the seventeenth day, the mitochondria have been supplied with **enzymes** that power the movement or contraction of the primitive myocardial cells, and the heart of the embryo has begun to beat. (The genetic and chemical processes controlling these amazingly rapid changes are now being studied in chick embryos and other models.)

Looping of the heart: looping defects

By the twenty-third day after conception the human embryo is 2.2 millimeters long. The heart tube now has four layers: the endocardium,
the myocardium, the cardiac jelly, and an outer layer of cells called
the **pericardium**. The heart now twists or loops toward the right (figure
2.5). This **looping** of the heart is under very strong genetic control;
only very occasionally does the loop go in the opposite direction.
When this happens we say that a looping defect is present. This is
the first thing that can go wrong in the fetus's developing heart (see
chapter 7).

By the time the embryo is five millimeters long (approximately
twenty-seven days) blood is already circulating from the heart to the
rest of the embryo, although the oxygen and nutrition needed for fetal
growth continue to come from the placenta, which will supply these
needs until the time of birth. The heart tube is now folding on itself.
The receiving chamber, or atrium, now lies nearer to the embryo's head
than does the pumping chamber, the primitive ventricle. The ventricle
leads into a large single vessel called the **truncus arteriosus**, or truncus, which later divides into two vessels, the aorta and the pulmonary
artery.

Cardiac jelly to endocardial cushions: endocardial cushion defects

The cardiac jelly becomes more elaborate and helps to form the **endocardial cushions** (figure 2.5). These cushions gradually thin out and
play an important part in forming the delicate yet tough heart valves
and part of both septa. In one serious form of heart defect, this jelly
does not separate properly: it seems somehow to have been wrongly
programmed. As a result, a complete atrioventricular canal remains in
the center of the heart. This canal is normal in embryos of about nine
millimeters or thirty days, but if still present at birth, it can cause much
difficulty. Such **atrioventricular canal defects** are frequent in Down
syndrome (see chapters 6 and 15).

The developing aorta and pulmonary artery: conotruncal defects

Some important cells have moved into the upper pole of the heart tube
from the primitive nervous system and the arches that form the head
and neck. These migrating ("neural crest") cells later take part in forming the connection between the heart and the lungs. At the same time
as the ventricles are beginning to separate, changes are taking place in

2.5. The Fetal Heart

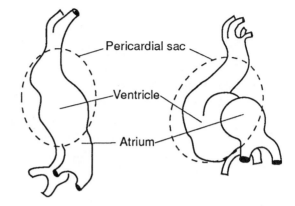

Looping. The primitive heart tube curves inside the pericardium, so that the apex of the heart, the future left ventricle, points to the left. When the looping process is disturbed, mirror image dextrocardia or other looping defects may occur.

Pericardial sac

Ventricle

Atrium

Endocardial cushions. When the embryo is 9-mm long, the endocardial cushions begin to form swellings that help in separating the atrioventricular canal and in forming the matrix or groundwork of the heart valves.

R. atrium

Endocardial cushions

L. atrium

Ventricle

Primitive atrioventricular canal surrounded by growing endocardial cushions

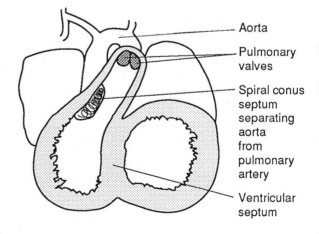

Conotruncal and ventricular septation. When the embryo is 16-mm long, the aorta and pulmonary artery have been separated by the spiral conotruncus septum, so that the right part of the ventricle leads to the pulmonary artery, the left to the aorta. The ventricular septum and atrial septum are still forming.

Illustrations by Edward B. Clark, M.D.

Aorta

Pulmonary valves

Spiral conus septum separating aorta from pulmonary artery

Ventricular septum

the truncus and in the area of the heart leading from the ventricle to the truncus. The changes in this **conotruncal area** are complicated and are still the subject of some argument. However, two important events are known to occur. First, a spiral wall or septum grows vertically in the conotruncus, separating it into two arteries, the aorta and the pulmonary artery (figure 2.5). These two arteries form by equal division and are approximately equal in size. Second, the artery to the lungs, or pulmonary artery, comes to lie in front of the aorta and to join the right ventricle. When this spiraling goes awry, a conotruncal defect is the result (see chapter 5).

Septation of the walls of the heart and development of the heart valves: septal defects and heart flow defects

Between the twenty-seventh and thirty-seventh days of development the two atria become separated by a wall, the atrial septum. However, this wall continues to have a small opening in it—called the **foramen ovale** because of its oval shape—and blood can pass between the atria until the time of birth. A wall grows between the ventricles, made up partly of muscle and partly of tissues coming from the cardiac jelly. The growth of the walls separating the right and left sides of the heart is called **septation**. Septal defects—failure of completion of the atrial or ventricular septum—are among the most common childhood heart problems (see chapter 4).

The aortic and pulmonary valves develop from endocardial cushion tissue as the truncus is dividing. At first the valves are little bumps or ridges in the truncus wall; then they thin out to become thin delicate valves, each with three cusps that meet perfectly as they close. These valves develop during the time that the embryo is growing from fourteen to forty millimeters in length, so they are still forming while most of the heart has already developed into the four chambers needed for life outside the womb.

The size of the two ventricles is critically important to life after birth. If the right ventricle is too small, not enough blood reaches the lungs. Even worse, if the left ventricle is too small, too little blood will reach the body. Our present understanding is that the two ventricles divide equally early in embryonic life, probably by seven weeks, when the embryo is fourteen to fifteen millimeters long. If something disturbs the normal flow of blood through the early heart, the growth of that particular chamber may be affected.

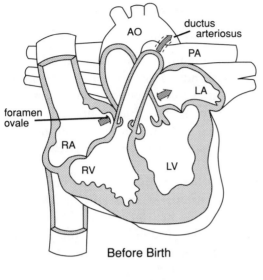

Before Birth

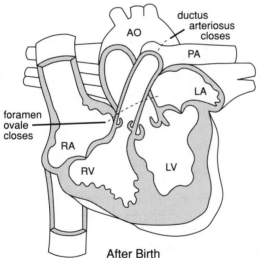

After Birth

2.6.
The Normal Heart before and after Birth

During life in the womb, the right ventricle is the dominant one. Most of the blood returning to the fetal heart bypasses the lungs, reaching the left ventricle through the hole in the atrial septum (the foramen ovale), or it passes from the pulmonary artery to the aorta through the ductus arteriosus (figure 2.6). The foramen ovale and the ductus arteriosus are important during life in the womb, but they normally close soon after birth.

Changes in the Heart

At birth

There are few moments in life more dramatic than an infant's first cry. No matter how often writers and movie directors have portrayed this moment, that unique and unforgettable sound retains its impact, for in that moment the baby takes on an independent life. The lungs, which have been quiescent although not inactive in the womb, are now essential to life. At that moment blood must begin to circulate efficiently throughout the lungs.

Several things happen together. As the breath goes in, the lungs expand with air and the pressure in the lungs falls, so blood can flow more easily into the lungs at the next heartbeat. After reaching the lungs, the blood returns to the left atrium, making the pressure higher on the left than on the right side of the atrial septum. The foramen ovale becomes unimportant and gradually seals shut.

Once the first breath has filled the lungs with air, the oxygen level in the infant's blood rises. This higher level of oxygen in the aorta causes the muscle in the wall of the ductus to contract in a kind of spasm, and no more blood flows through the ductus. Although the ductus has played an important role in circulation during life in the womb, that role is now over. If the ductus stays open, as it occasionally does (especially in premature babies), it can delay the newborn's adaptation to life outside the womb. A ductus that remains open is called a patent ductus arteriosus, often abbreviated PDA.

With growth

Changes in the circulation with growth vary from the simple and well known to the complex. Best known are the changes in heart rate. In general, the heart rate of a newborn baby will vary from an average of about 110 beats per minute when the baby is asleep to 180 beats per minute when the baby is active or feeding. A healthy 10-year-old will have a resting heart rate of 80 to 100 beats per minute, rising to 180 with exercise. The rate of increase in heart rate with exercise will depend at least partly on the level of fitness of the child and in any case will be less abrupt than in a newborn. An athletic, muscular adolescent may have a resting pulse rate of 60 to 80, which will rise to 180 or 200 only after quite prolonged strenuous exercise.

Blood pressure rises slowly with growth. A **systolic blood pressure** of seventy millimeters of mercury and a **diastolic blood pressure** of 50 millimeters of mercury (70/50 mm Hg) is normal in a healthy newborn; 100/70 mm Hg would be normal in a healthy teenager.

The heart itself grows as the child grows. The actual size of the heart chambers increases, as does the thickness of the muscle wall or myocardium.

Messages pass continually between the brain and heart, messages that help to control the rate of the heart and its response to changes in the surroundings. As the child grows, the network of nerves and nerve endings that pass on these messages becomes more complex and sophisticated; some of the chemical interactions also change. During childhood, the walls of the arteries become thicker and slightly less resilient or elastic, but severe changes in the arteries seldom occur.

The changes in circulation with growth are designed to keep up with the child's needs. The tissues of a child weighing eighty pounds must be supplied with larger amounts of oxygen than those of an infant weighing ten pounds. The slowing of the heart rate and the increase in size of the heart chambers make possible an increase in cardiac output, that is, the quantity of blood put out by each heartbeat. An older child can deliver more oxygen and nutrition to the body with each heartbeat than an infant can. Anyone who has watched the inexhaustible energy of a healthy 10-year-old has seen good cardiac output in action!

The Sounds of the Normal Heart

As the heart pumps blood into the body, two sounds are produced. The first, a thudding sound caused by the contraction of the heart muscle, is easy to hear with a stethoscope or even by applying an ear to the chest wall. The second heart sound, more difficult to hear, occurs when the aortic and pulmonary valves close after blood has been pumped out to the body and lungs. (The lub-dup, lub-dup sounds [figure 2.7] can be reproduced on tape recordings, and are often used in programs on radio and television.) Extra sounds between lub and dup are known as "heart murmurs." In conditions in which the heartbeat is weak, there may be heart failure or cardiomyopathy. If the heart rhythm is disturbed, as in arrhythmias, the lub and dup occur erratically.

Congenital and Acquired Heart Problems

The normal heart grows and develops from a single tube to a highly efficient four-chambered structure that is exquisitely responsive to the

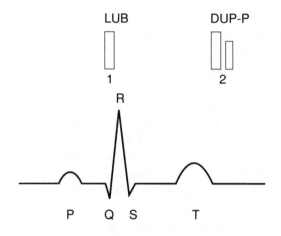

2.7. Heart Sounds and Electrocardiogram. The first heart sound, *LUB*, occurs when the ventricle contracts: the second sound, *DUP-P*, is produced by closure of the aortic, and a little later, of the pulmonary valve. On the electrocardiogram, *shown below*, the P wave occurs as the atrium contracts, the QRS complex as the ventricle contracts, and the T wave as electrical repolarization of the heart occurs during ventricular relaxation (diastole).

needs of the growing child. If, however, the heart develops abnormally in the womb, the child may be born with a congenital heart defect. Later in the book we will give examples of how different congenital heart defects can be treated and how most children with these defects can be restored to normal health.

In other children the heart develops normally in the womb, but after birth the muscle or valves of the heart may be damaged by an infection such as rheumatic fever or a viral inflammation of the heart muscle (viral myocarditis). In yet other children, an arrhythmia is present—the normal, regular rhythm of the heart is lost. Most such heart problems appearing after birth (**acquired heart disease**) also can be successfully treated.

The majority of childhood heart problems are a consequence of some abnormality of development before birth. In the next chapter we will review some of the risk factors for congenital heart defects. As soon as parents hear of the possibility that their infant may have been born with any heart defect, however mild, they ask *Why?*

Chapter 3

The Risk Factors for Heart Defects

Almost all heart defects can now be treated and most can be treated successfully, many in early infancy. But no statistics and no diagram can describe the effect on a family when they learn their baby has a heart defect, severe or mild. Doctors still cannot answer all the questions that are of passionate interest to patients and their families:

- "Why our child?"
- "Why didn't anyone warn us?"
- "Is it our fault?"
- "How did it happen?"

When a family turns to us for answers to these questions, most of the time we have only meager information. Usually we cannot pinpoint the exact cause of the defect in the child's heart. Even when a certain defect is known to be associated with (that is, to coexist frequently with) a specific chromosomal disorder, gaps still remain in our knowledge of how and why this is so. For example, we still do not know for certain why endocardial cushion defects are fifty times more common in children with Down syndrome than in children who have normal chromosomes (see chapter 15).

In trying to track down causes, scientists have looked for predisposing risk factors in children and their families. Dr. Charlotte Ferencz, director of the Baltimore-Washington Infant Study (BWIS) of heart defects in babies, has likened the search to working a gigantic jigsaw puzzle. Pieces of knowledge are gradually accumulated and then fitted together, carefully and sometimes laboriously, to form a picture.

One way of thinking about causes is to ask what is different about a child with a heart defect. The development of the heart is extremely complicated, yet more than 99 babies in 100 are born with no heart defect at all. What happens to make that 1 baby out of 100 different? Is it Nature—some genetic abnormality? Or is it Nurture—some toxin or other influence in the environment? We know, for example, that certain drugs—such as thalidomide or isoretinoic acid—can damage the developing heart, and that if a mother has **rubella** (German measles) early in pregnancy, the baby's heart and other organs may develop abnormally. Is it perhaps a combination of both—can a drug or toxin affect one embryonic heart and not another because of genetic differences? Or does the defect simply occur by chance? So many genes and biochemical pathways are involved in the growth of the heart from a primitive tube to a complex four-chambered organ that it is easy to believe that a chance happening could sometimes lead to error. Dr. Helen Taussig, the pioneering cardiologist, wrote late in her career that the similarity of heart defects in birds, animals, and humans suggests that some defects occurred early in the evolution of each species. Scientists must continue to look for causes and patterns.

It is vital to remember that the search for causes is not the search for fault or blame. Chance may play a role in heart defects, as in everything we do. In fact, seven times out of ten we have no clue to the cause of heart defects in particular persons.

As soon as a heart defect is diagnosed parents are overwhelmed by specific questions and doubts. Does one of the parents carry a faulty gene? Could the defect have been prevented? Did one parent inadvertently expose the tiny developing heart to some toxic agent? Parents agonize over such questions. Almost always we can reassure them that they did nothing to cause the problem. Families' interest in risk factors, quite naturally, often far surpasses that of many physicians and health workers.

A number of different approaches to the study of risk factors have been used. One of the oldest and simplest methods is to look carefully at families that have more than one person with a heart defect. These studies of familial aggregations have shown clearly that genetic risk factors are important. Doppler-echocardiography can now be used to prove or disprove the presence of mild defects in apparently healthy family members. Some of the sophisticated tools of modern geneticists are now being applied to the study of such families. Within the next two decades many of the genes responsible for severe defects will have been mapped. Other studies of risk factors are epidemiologic studies, animal studies, and embryologic studies. Studies also have considered the risk to the fetus of various environmental risks and of illnesses of the mother, as well as the effect of chemicals, medications, female sex hormones, drugs, caffeine, alcohol, and tobacco used by the mother.

Studies of Risk Factors: How We Know What Little We Know

Epidemiologic studies

Epidemiologic studies—including the BWIS, in which the authors participated—compare details of the family history and pregnancy exposures of parents and infants born with normal and with abnormal hearts. The great advantage of such studies is that they are representative of the population as a whole, and thus comparative studies of differences in toxic exposure or in family history between children with heart defects and those who are healthy are not biased in any way. When an exposure to maternal illness is very rare, however, not enough mothers will be included to permit sound conclusions to be drawn. No one type of study has all the answers.

Epidemiologic studies showed many years ago that Down syndrome was more likely to occur in infants of older than of younger mothers; that is, older maternal age was shown to be a risk factor for Down syndrome. The BWIS and other cardiac studies now are focusing on family history, on medications taken during pregnancy, and on work exposures as risk factors for heart defects.

Animal studies

Animal studies have been used to analyze genetic factors in heart defects; it is known that certain breeds of dog—poodles, for example—are more likely to have a patent ductus arteriosus than are other breeds. It is possible to study genetic factors by selective inbreeding for such a defect. In teratologic studies, drugs or toxins are given to pregnant animals to gain useful information on the tendency of the drug or toxin to cause heart or other defects. Such studies have limitations, because different animals may react differently to drugs. For example, thalidomide did not damage the hearts of embryo rabbits, but it did damage the human fetal heart. Nonetheless, much valuable knowledge can be learned and many human tragedies prevented through animal studies. For example, for many years researchers have maintained a special mouse colony characterized by looping defects of the heart; recently an abnormal gene has been identified as causing these defects.

Embryologic studies

These studies of normal animal hearts are now quite advanced. Studies of how the chick heart rate and blood pressure change with growth, and of how normal development can be affected by drugs or temperature, for example, have added considerably to our understanding of the more complex human heart. The chick circulatory system can also be studied more completely than can the circulation of other animals. A chick is very different from a child, but early in their development many animals, including humans, have certain developmental stages in common.

This is an extraordinarily active and dynamic period in knowledge of heart development. Although we do not yet know enough to ensure that each child will be born with a normal heart, the remarkable processes involved in the development of the healthy, growing heart and the processes that lead to problems in the heart are beginning to be understood.

Genetic Risk Factors

One of the great family joys of having a new baby is looking for likenesses. Is his chin like his father's? Are her eyes the soft gray-blue of her mother's? Does he really favor his grandfather? We have all played these happy, inconclusive guessing games of recognition and memory. But when a heart defect is found in an infant, the questions may be very different and may be a source of stress and tension. One father asked:

> *Why does little Matthew have this heart defect? Mary and I planned so carefully for him. I knew when we married that Mary's family had had a lot of heart attacks; in fact, her brother Dick, who is only 40, is in intensive care right now. We've never had anything like that in my family. Do you think there's some connection there? What are our chances of ever having a healthy baby?*

The problem in Matthew's heart cannot be "blamed" on Mary's

family. We know positively that there is no connection between heart attacks in adults and heart defects in newborn infants.

Mendelian syndromes

In a few families, certain heart defects do indeed pass from one generation to the next. The family may have a Mendelian syndrome. **Syndrome** (*syn* = join, *drome* = run together) means a cluster of defects or problems that are often seen together.

Mendelian inheritance is named after Gregor Mendel, author of the modern study of genetics. If a defect or syndrome is expressed in one generation after another it is said to show an "autosomal dominant" mode of inheritance. This means that the gene is carried not on the X or Y chromosomes (the sex chromosomes), but on one of the other ("autosomal") chromosomes.

> *Ella R. was found to have a heart murmur when she was 2. She was otherwise healthy and active. After the cardiologist had examined her and had performed some tests, including an EKG and an echo-Doppler, he told the parents that Ella had an atrial septal defect; that is, the wall or septum between her right and left atria was incomplete. The cardiologist asked if anyone else in the family had any congenital defects. Mrs. R., the mother, held out her left hand: the thumb was missing. A little embarrassed because he had not noticed this before, the cardiologist now looked more closely at Ella's tiny hands; her thumbs looked more like fingers than thumbs.*
>
> *After consulting with a geneticist and obtaining some additional family history, the cardiologist concluded that atrial septal defect and hand abnormalities were clearly inherited on the mother's side of the family, varying in severity between one family member and another.*

Mrs. R's family had an abnormal gene for Holt-Oram syndrome, one of a number of syndromes in which heart and hand go together.

In other Mendelian syndromes the single gene may be silent: each parent is carrying an abnormal gene although each parent appears quite normal. One of their infants may receive a double dose of the abnormal gene—one gene from each parent—and develop a disease or a defect. Such recessive modes of inheritance occur, for example, in cystic fibrosis and sickle cell anemia. Virtually all looping defects of the heart are inherited this way.

Mendelian syndromes are rare, accounting for only about 1 percent of all septal or conotruncal defects. Nevertheless, they are involved in about 5 percent of **right-heart flow defects** in infants and in virtually all looping defects. Parents will want to discuss with their physician the possibility of such a single-gene syndrome if their baby has more than one defect in addition to the heart defect, or if other members of the family have major congenital defects.

Down syndrome (trisomy 21) and other chromosomal syndromes

Because genes are carried on the chromosomes, it is not surprising that when the infant's chromosomes are abnormal in number or arrangement a greatly increased risk of a heart defect exists. However, chromosomal defects do not usually "run in the family." An infant with Down syndrome has three copies of chromosome 21 (trisomy 21) rather than the normal pair; this extra chromosome leads to many abnormalities, including heart defects in almost half of such infants. Endocardial cushion defects are particularly common in infants with Down syndrome (60 percent of infants with endocardial cushion defects have this syndrome); septal defects and tetralogy occur more rarely. Twelve percent of infants born with heart defects also have a chromosomal syndrome.

An infant with Turner syndrome (also called XO syndrome) is a female, but she is lacking the second X chromosome found in normal females; almost one-third of such infants have **left-heart flow defects**.

In the BWIS, 12 percent of infants under 1 year of age who were diagnosed as having heart defects had significant chromosomal abnormalities, the most frequent being Down syndrome. Perhaps even more important, more than 60 percent of all infants in that study who had endocardial cushion defects also had Down syndrome. This knowledge gives hope that new information about chromosome 21 will help infants who have both endocardial cushion defects and Down syndrome.

Other syndromes

Most other syndromes do not recur in families. Sometimes an infant is born with defects not only in the heart but in other organs. Such syndromes—that is, the occurrence of the same cluster of defects in many babies—may hold important clues for our future understanding of how different parts of the body develop, and of how one toxin or a single gene can affect many organs. The genetic implications of such syndromes still need study, and most families of infants with such problems should receive individual counselling from both a cardiologist and a geneticist. Parents of a child with a syndrome often feel frustrated and anxious, as each day seems to bring news of yet another problem. A coordinating primary-care nurse or physician and enrollment in a family support group can help make the future more manageable and hopeful.

Most babies with a heart defect do not have a syndrome. Everything except the heart is normal. In three babies out of four, or 75 percent of the time, the heart defect is the only problem—what geneticists call an "isolated" defect. Young parents will, of course, want to know how likely it is that any child born later will have a normal heart.

Genetic Risk Factors in Isolated Heart Defects

Many studies over the years have shown that only about 4 percent of the siblings of children with isolated heart defects will themselves have heart defects. If a sibling does have a heart defect, about six times out of ten it will be the same kind the brother or sister has.

Another way of saying this is that of 200 brothers and sisters of children born with a ventricular septal defect, 192 will have normal hearts and 8 will have heart defects. Of those eight, five will have ventricular septal defects. The knowledge that most siblings will have normal hearts is very reassuring to families. Some of the happiest letters and photographs we receive from parents come at Christmastime. One such photograph showed little Michael, who had had heart surgery as an infant and is now a "terrible 2," together with his healthy new baby sister, Jennifer, born with a normal heart.

Does the risk to the next baby, sometimes called by the rather forbidding term "sibling recurrence risk," of about 4 percent apply to all groups of isolated defects? A recent important family study has shown that isolated left-heart flow defects are more likely than any other group to run in a family. Using careful family histories and confirming any suspicious heart findings with echo-Doppler testing, the investigators found that 10 to 15 percent of siblings or parents of children with left-heart flow defects had heart abnormalities. The relative's abnormality also usually involved left-heart flow, but often it was much milder than in the original patient. Such families have about a three times higher risk of recurrence than families with other types of defects, a risk close to that found with recessive syndromes. This is all very important new information and is being studied further. (Some illustra-

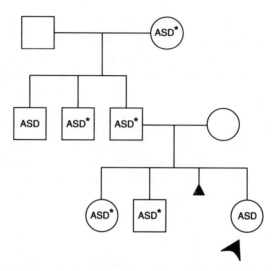

3.1. Inheritance of Atrial Septal Defect. In this and other family diagrams, males are shown by *squares,* females by *circles,* and the *arrow* indicates the original, or index, patient (the person first seen by the physician). A *black triangle* indicates a pregnancy ending in spontaneous abortion. *Key: ASD =* atrial septal defect; * = hand anomaly.

In this family with Holt-Oram syndrome, ASD and hand anomalies are seen in three generations and in both males and females. This pattern is typical of a Mendelian syndrome with autosomal dominant inheritance. The father of the index patient has a 40- to 50-percent chance that any subsequent baby will have an atrial septal defect and/or hand abnormality. There is thought to be an abnormality of a single gene, or perhaps a cluster of genes close together on the same chromosome.

tive family trees are shown in figures 3.1 and 3.2.)

The genes that influence flow through the left side of the heart in the embryo are presently unknown. New family studies are under way to look for these genes and to analyze why some family members have a mild defect such as a bicuspid aortic valve and others a severe life-threatening problem such as a **hypoplastic** left ventricle (see chapter 4).

Environmental Risk Factors

Parents of a child with a heart defect often ask themselves what caused this defect. Was it water pollution? A medicine I took? Something I ate? An illness I had? Since Rachel Carson published her influential

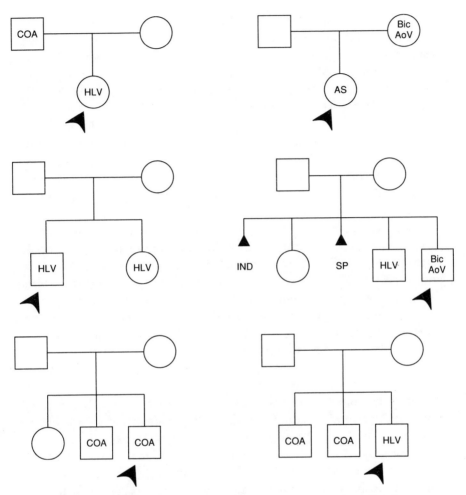

3.2. Familial Left-Sided Lesions with Varying Severity. In these family trees, you can see how both severe and milder left-heart flow defects can occur in the same family. In the family on the top left, a father who had been successfully operated on for aortic coarctation had a baby girl with hypoplastic left ventricle. *Key: COA* = coarctation of the aorta; *AS* = aortic valve stenosis; *Bic AoV* = bicuspid aortic valve; *HLV* = hypoplastic left ventricle; *SP* = spontaneous abortion; *IND* = induced abortion.

book *Silent Spring* in 1956, we have all become sensitive to the hazards of pollution and the toxins that surround us. Some drugs or toxins may damage the embryo heart, but the consistent rates and types of heart defects among people of many different countries, with their differing diets and customs, suggest that environment plays a relatively small role in causing most heart defects.

As the heart of the child forms in the embryo in the mother's womb, it lives in a special microenvironment or microcosm of its own. There the heart beats and grows, protected from many of the dangers of the outside world. But that microcosm is to a great extent controlled by the mother, by what she eats and drinks, and even perhaps by an illness she may have.

What can endanger that tiny enclosed world where a new heart is forming, a new life beginning? It would take more than one large book to review all the drugs and agents studied that may cross the placenta and reach the infant's heart. The most vulnerable period for the heart, the time when a toxic agent is most able to produce a malformation, is between fourteen and sixty days after conception, the time when the heart is forming, changing from a simple tube to a beating heart with four chambers and delicate yet sturdy valves.

Radiation

Radiation has much more effect on the developing brain than on the heart. Still, enormous radiation doses of 100 rads or more (equivalent to 12,500 chest X-rays) can produce heart defects in experimental animals, although there is no evidence at present that radiation is the cause of heart defects in human infants. Diagnostic X-rays during pregnancy are to be avoided unless required for the mother's own health. Careful continuous monitoring of exposure of everyone who works with radiation is essential.

Microwave radiation and exposure to electromagnetic fields have no proven relationship to heart defects.

Illness of the mother

Although most pregnant women are young and healthy, a cold or viral illness may occur at some time during the approximately forty weeks of pregnancy. The placenta, that remarkable structure that supplies oxygen, minerals, and everything necessary for the baby's growth, can also pass on viruses. Viruses are the proven cause of heart defects in about 2 percent of infants with these defects.

The rubella (German measles) epidemics of 1940 and 1964 brought viral illness to the world's attention. The rubella virus was shown to cross the placenta and, depending on the time in pregnancy, cause damage to the fetal heart, brain, and eyes. The role of other viruses is not so clear and has been difficult to study. Heart defects do not seem to increase nine months after influenza epidemics, for example, and no real variation with seasons or infections has been proven.

Arrhythmias and even heart failure in the fetus and newborn can be caused by a virus. If a mother develops a Coxsackie virus infection late in pregnancy, the infant may be born with myocarditis or, perhaps, heart failure as a consequence of inflammation of the heart muscle (see chapter 8). But this virus is not known to cause malformations of the heart, as rubella does.

The AIDS virus (human immunodeficiency virus, or HIV) also can invade the fetal heart and cause myocarditis and heart failure; it is suspected of having been the cause of heart defects in a few infants, but this is uncertain. Cytomegalovirus, toxoplasmosis, and certain other viruses that may lead to deafness or mental retardation rarely if ever cause heart defects.

At present no virus other than rubella is clearly associated with any specific heart defect.

In the BWIS, mothers of infants who had heart defects and mothers whose infants had none were equally likely to have had cold and flu symptoms during pregnancy. However, the taking of antibiotics during pregnancy was shown to be a mild risk factor for heart defects. Although it is extremely difficult to separate medications from the reason they were taken, particularly in studies involving recall of what happened nine to twelve months previously, at present it seems that ordinary respiratory illnesses play a minor role in causing heart defects, if they play any role at all.

An illness in the mother such as **diabetes** always causes concern about complications during pregnancy. There is also concern about how the illness may affect the developing heart. Diabetic mothers, particularly those who need ongoing treatment with insulin, are three times more likely than nondiabetics to have an infant with a heart defect. Severe or insulin-dependent diabetes is a major risk factor for conotruncal defects, especially ones of double outlet right ventricle and truncus arteriosus (see chapter 5). When diabetes develops late in pregnancy and disappears after the baby is born (gestational diabetes), however, there seems to be less risk of a heart defect in the baby.

Babies of heavy birth weight born to diabetic mothers may have enlarged hearts after birth because of thickening of the heart muscle (hypertrophic cardiomyopathy). Fortunately, this condition disappears over the next few weeks.

> *I am 30 years old and have two healthy children—Jane, aged 5, and Joshua, aged 2. I have been on oral medication for diabetes for the past year. I am now sixteen weeks pregnant and my doctor says I am fine. Are you saying I will have a "blue baby"?*

This mother is in the group of "mild" diabetics who do not need insulin. Her risk of having a baby with some type of heart problem is about twice the usual risk; nevertheless, her baby has a 98-percent likelihood of having a normal heart. Keeping her blood sugar as close to normal as possible is good for the baby's heart and for her own long-term health. Good control of the diabetes itself is important, even if this requires some extra laboratory tests and clinical visits. Enrolling in a support group composed of young diabetic mothers may be helpful for her peace of mind. This mother's obstetrician probably will recommend a fetal echocardiogram in about the 20th week of pregnancy to monitor the development of the baby's heart.

Epilepsy in the mother seems to have only a very slight effect on the fetal heart unless the mother is receiving phenytoin (Dilantin) treatment, in which case she has three to five times the usual risk of having an infant with a heart defect. Different studies have not agreed on the risk. The differing conclusions may be caused by the fact that some people metabolize phenytoin more slowly than others; also, one study may have included more slow metabolizers than others. It is clear that certain other minor defects, including short fingernails and some developmental delay, are much more common than heart defects in the children of mothers who take phenytoin. This phenytoin syndrome is an important reason for a young woman of childbearing age who has epilepsy to discuss with her physician whether anticonvulsants are still necessary before she becomes pregnant.

If additional anticonvulsant drugs are needed, the risk is further increased, particularly in the case of trimethadione. Because seizure control may be vital for the mother's health and safety, individual review is needed *before* she becomes pregnant. Increasingly often, a mother who needed medication to control seizures in early childhood is found to have outgrown that need, thus improving her chance of having a healthy baby. Antiepileptic drugs increase the risk of both conotruncal and septal defects.

Systemic lupus erythematosus (SLE) is a rare disorder, one of a family of autoimmune diseases in which the mother produces antibodies against her own tissue. SLE in the mother seldom if ever causes any of the usual heart defects discussed later in this book; however, in a mother with SLE, substances known as Ro antibodies may cross the placenta and cause fibrous scar tissue to form around the developing conducting system in the embryo's heart. This scar tissue results in an excessively slow heart rate and abnormal rhythm, known as complete **heart block**. Not all babies of mothers with SLE are affected, however, and a great deal of research is now under way to determine why some babies have natural protection and how to protect the others.

Phenylketonuria, or PKU, a rare and severe problem of childhood, has been treated successfully by diet for many years, allowing many patients to reach adulthood. However, if a young pregnant woman with PKU still has high levels of phenylalanine in her blood, this will damage the infant's developing heart and brain. Full reevaluation is essential *before* starting a pregnancy, and the future mother needs to be on a special diet, low in phenylalanine,

Illnesses that have not been shown to cause heart defects include thyroid disorders, high fever (hyperthermia), and hypertension. In the BWIS familial blood disorders were found to be associated statistically with a slight increase in infant heart defects, but it was an association too slight to be of concern to any particular family.

Chemicals

We are all alive and functioning normally because of a remarkable balance of essential chemicals in our own bodies and in our surroundings. But are there chemicals that can damage the developing heart?

Industrial and environmental chemicals remain a subject of great public concern. A number of substances used in industry, including mercury, lead, thallium, and lithium, can damage an embryo if given in very high concentration in the feed or drinking water of a pregnant animal. None of these chemicals has been shown to affect the hearts of infants whose parents have been exposed to them in the modern workplace, where occupational toxins are now carefully controlled. Lead exposure from paint stripping and other home activities is currently being studied as a possible risk factor for a small number of mothers.

In a few studies, mothers working as anesthetists have been shown to have a slightly increased risk of having an infant with a heart defect. Other agents studied, including hair spray used by beauticians, hexachlorophene used in soap by nurses, pesticides, and exposure of the *father* to high-voltage electrical fields, have shown no consistent pattern.

Medications

Medications have been studied intensively as possible risk factors since 1962, when it was recognized that thalidomide, used in many countries as a sedative, produced tragic fetal deformities if taken by a mother in early pregnancy. The drug caused severe limb defects known as phocomelia, in which arms or legs were replaced by little seal-like flippers. Heart defects, although less common, were also severe; these defects were chiefly conotruncal abnormalities resembling tetralogy. This drug is now banned.

Isotretinoic acid (Accutane), a drug effective in the treatment of acne and severe skin diseases, has been shown, like thalidomide, to cross the placenta and to cause serious conotruncal defects of the heart and abnormal development of the nervous system in the developing fetus. It therefore should not be used by young women of childbearing age.

Sex hormones have been intensively studied as possible risk factors. Investigations in the 1960s suggested that the female sex hormones estrogen and progesterone (the two principal components of birth control pills and used in various combinations in the management of infertility and gynecologic disorders) increased the risk of heart defects in infants, especially the risk of tetralogy or transposition if the hormones were used around the time of conception. Other studies were started, but at the same time the dose of hormones being used in treatment was in the process of being reduced. The consensus is that these drugs are now minimally, if at all, involved in causing heart defects. Nevertheless, if such medications can be discontinued before a woman attempts to become pregnant, this should be done.

Psychotropic drugs may need to be continued during pregnancy to allow the mother to remain a functional member of society. Lithium, useful in manic-depressive illness, does increase the risk of a heart defect in the infant, perhaps as much as ten times, but the risk may need to be taken. However, phenothiazine, a frequently prescribed tranquilizer, doubles the risk of a heart defect and should be avoided if possible.

Of the many other drugs in the class, including diazepam (Valium), chlordiazepoxide (Librium), and a growing number of others, none is clearly implicated in producing heart defects. Yet every study involving infants with and without defects has shown psychotropic drugs to be a risk factor, although a mild and inconclusive one. A careful review of the benefits of (and need for) the medication should be undertaken before a woman embarks on pregnancy.

A large number of other prescription medications have been investigated but have not clearly been shown to cause heart defects. Anthracyclines and drugs used to treat childhood cancer are capable of producing birth defects in animals but have not been found to increase the risk of heart defects in infants.

Bendectin, once frequently used to prevent nausea and morning sickness, is now off the market. Multiple studies have not shown it to cause heart defects.

Nonprescription medications, or over-the-counter drugs, can be found in the medicine chest of almost every household. The average young American woman takes 1.3 such medications during pregnancy, in addition to prescribed iron and vitamins. At least one-third of pregnant women take none of these drugs, however, and fewer such drugs are ingested now than in the 1960s. Dr. Judy Rubin and her colleagues in the BWIS have discovered these encouraging trends; she is continuing to analyze what new conclusions and advice should come from the study.

Aspirin taken in large doses in early pregnancy was found in one study to double the risk of a heart defect, but other studies have not confirmed this.

> *If everyone takes all these pills, how do we know they do any harm? Every time I get a cold my sinuses act up; I get a headache "this big" and a runny nose. I always take product XYZ for my colds. Why shouldn't I take it now I'm five weeks pregnant?*

No one can really answer these questions with certainty. Drugs such as aspirin and some cold medicines were around long before testing in pregnancy was even thought of, and there is no proof they harm the developing heart. We do know three things that may help in personal decisions: (1) Almost all drugs cross the placenta; this means they reach the baby. (2) No drug is known to improve heart development. (3) No drug is known to protect from heart defects. We strongly recommend that the mother avoid all unnecessary self-medication in pregnancy, since the baby will get the medication, too.

Drugs of personal habit

I have always drunk about three cups of coffee a day. Will this affect my baby's heart?

I smoked cigarettes all during my pregnancy, only half a pack a day. My baby had an abnormal heart rhythm right after birth. That couldn't come from cigarettes, could it?

My daughter is a binge drinker, just like my husband. I'm sure she drank while she was carrying little Jo, although she says she didn't. Is this why Jo has a hole in her heart?

I smoked some pot at a party a few days before I knew I was pregnant. My boyfriend smokes it all the time. Our baby Jimmy has just died after heart surgery. I feel terrible, like it was all our fault. What do you think?

These are not just requests for scientific information. They involve the feelings of guilt and grief that are part of all serious illness; they are particularly poignant when the illness is that of a newborn infant. Drugs of personal habit range widely from the almost ubiquitous caffeine through alcohol to street drugs in various combinations.

Caffeine is in widespread use in coffee, tea, and chocolate. No increased risk of heart or other defects has been found with a consumption of caffeine equivalent to between one and three cups of coffee a day.

An enormous amount of research has been done on alcohol consumption during pregnancy, particularly in relation to brain development. In fetal alcohol syndrome there is severe retardation of physical and mental growth; facial abnormalities are common, and septal defects are found in the hearts of about 40 percent of such infants. Alcohol consumption by the pregnant woman only rarely causes conotruncal or other severe heart defects.

Atrial and ventricular septal defects are common in all countries and all cultures, and they certainly occur in infants of Seventh Day Adventists and other parents who never use alcohol. Although alcohol is not the *only* cause of septal defects, and although there is no evidence a single cocktail early in pregnancy can harm the fetal heart, heavy alcohol use does increase the risk of heart and brain problems, perhaps as much as forty times.

Particularly now that habits of lifestyle, such as cigarette smoking and drinking alcohol, are known to have major effects on long-term health in individuals and in populations, there is great concern about possible harm to the embryo and fetus from such habits. This is a difficult subject on which to gather information, and the question of harm can be answered only by careful epidemiologic studies.

Cocaine, marijuana, and heroin have not been conclusively shown to cause heart defects. One recent study that compared newborn babies who tested positive for cocaine with those drug-free at birth, however, found heart defects to be at least four times more frequent in babies who had been exposed to cocaine in the womb. Another study of infants of mothers with heavy cocaine use showed many defects in the heart and other parts of the body, some probably due to damage to the blood supply of the brain, the intestines, and other organs. We know that cocaine is very toxic to the adult heart, causing spasm of the coronary arteries, and it has caused fatal arrhythmias and sudden death even in some healthy athletes. All these drugs slow the growth of the infant in the womb. Heroin and crack cocaine can also affect the adult heart, causing abnormal heart rhythms and even sudden death. No studies have shown that these drugs cause heart defects, but parents who use these illegal drugs cannot care properly for any child, whether healthy or with a heart problem.

Common sense and love of the unborn child strongly urge against exposing the defenseless fetus to such toxins.

Smoking of tobacco by the mother can slow growth of the infant before birth but has not been shown to cause heart defects or to cause abnormal heart rhythms in the baby. However, cigarette smoking is unhealthy for everyone in the family.

The Role of Chance

About seven times out of ten we can find no clue to the cause of a heart defect. The baby is otherwise normal and we have to assume that some transient disturbance affected the growth of the heart at a critical time. Chance seems to be involved in most septal defects, for example, although we know that the risk of septal defects is increased by the mother's use of alcohol and certain other drugs. With further research the role of chance will be seen to diminish. As more elaborate methods are used to analyze family data, the role of genetic factors is increasingly recognized. Even in the commonest defect of all, the small ventricular septal defect, we may find that there is a familial predisposition. Genetic factors are particularly important in some syndromes and in left-heart flow defects.

Figure 3.3, a schematic drawing of an embryo, shows some of the risk factors which have been studied.

The concept of risk factors for the developing heart is similar to that for atherosclerosis. Just as high blood **cholesterol** is not "the cause" of atherosclerosis but a major risk factor, so the chromosomal abnormality of Down syndrome is the single major risk factor for, but not the sole cause of, endocardial cushion defect.

As the painstaking search for risk factors and causes continues, a difficult balance must be maintained between an ardent pursuit of new clues and a recognition that the overwhelming number of infants—99 out of 100—are born with normal hearts. As more is learned, we will be able to protect the developing heart even better than we can now, and heart defects will be seen far less frequently.

Will it happen again?

While we continue to search for better understanding of the heart and the prevention of heart defects, it remains true that in almost all families *nothing they did or did not do caused the defect*. In families with no other affected family members, and with no risk factors such as diabetes or drug use, the next child will have a normal heart about 95 percent of the time.

The risk of recurrence is higher when the family's infant has a looping or left-heart flow defect. If more than one family member has such a defect, or if the infant has a syndrome, study and genetic counselling may be needed.

> *Shelley has had surgery to close her ventricular septal defect. She is running around and seems fine. John and I have always wanted a second child. I took Librium and later some Valium while I was carrying Shelley. Should we have any extra tests before we plan another baby?*

Although Shelley and her parents have been through an ordeal, the future is now bright; Shelley should grow to be a healthy adult. In the absence of any risk factors, the next baby has at least 95 chances out of 100 of having a normal heart.

An echocardiogram of the fetus will not necessarily reveal a tiny defect in the ventricular septum, but it can be very reassuring for the

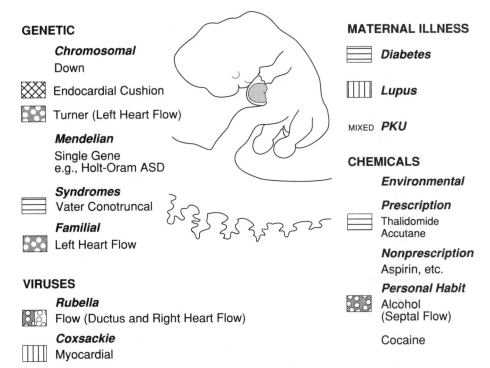

GENETIC

Chromosomal
Down

Endocardial Cushion

Turner (Left Heart Flow)

Mendelian
Single Gene
e.g., Holt-Oram ASD

Syndromes
Vater Conotruncal

Familial
Left Heart Flow

VIRUSES

Rubella
Flow (Ductus and Right Heart Flow)

Coxsackie
Myocardial

MATERNAL ILLNESS

Diabetes

Lupus

MIXED **PKU**

CHEMICALS

Environmental

Prescription
Thalidomide
Accutane

Nonprescription
Aspirin, etc.

Personal Habit
Alcohol
(Septal Flow)

Cocaine

3.3. Risk Factors and Heart Defects. Some risk factors that may affect the embryo heart include Down syndrome for endocardial cushion defect (shown by *cross-hatched symbol* as in figure 4.1), diabetes for conotruncal defects (*horizontal bars*), and rubella for flow defects (*circles* or *bubbles*). Although much still needs to be learned, in this chapter and the next we illustrate how defects and risk factors can be grouped in ways that make sense in light of our current knowledge.

parents of an earlier child with a heart defect to see that all four chambers of the heart are developing well. The fear of a seriously defective heart can be alleviated. Some families may find the following outline and checklist helpful as they prepare for their next baby.

Planning for the Next Baby

This outline plan may be considered a good general guide for a couple who have a child with a heart problem and are planning another pregnancy.

- Check general health with your doctor
- Review any special risk factors

- Check close family members (siblings and parents) for heart and other defects
- Register early for good obstetric care
- Begin optimal diet, weight, and exercise program
- Avoid alcohol, drugs, and all nonessential medications
- Arrange for a fetal cardiac echo test in the eighteenth to twentieth week of pregnancy

Using the following checklist for parents who have a child with a heart defect, you can confer with the physician and decide together if the outline plan above applies to you, or if extra tests or precautions are needed.

1. Do we know exactly what defect our baby has?   Y __ N __
2. What is the defect called?   _____
3. Which group of defects?   _____
4. Does the baby have any problems other than the heart defect? Y __ N __
5. If other defects are present, what are they? (Most defects, even obvious ones such as an extra finger, do not affect your next child's risk of a heart defect. But if there are several defects or a family syndrome, you may need a special individual conference with a skilled geneticist.)   _____
6. Do I, my family, or my husband's family have any special risk factors?   Y __ N __

May your next baby be born with the wonderful gift of a healthy heart!

Part II

HEART PROBLEMS IN CHILDREN

Chapter 4

Defects in the Developing Heart

During the months inside the mother's womb, the embryo has developed into a fetus that gradually becomes capable of sustaining life outside the womb. During early embryonic life, the heart develops into a remarkably complex four-chambered structure. In most people it will continue to beat rhythmically and effectively for many, many years. Sometimes, however, the heart has not developed as it should, and when the baby is born, its heart is in some way imperfect. The baby has a congenital heart defect.

"Defect" is an alarming word for a parent to hear. Every person on earth has some imperfections, but because the heart is a vital organ for sustaining life, the very mention of a heart defect can arouse in parents great anxiety and even panic. Even though heart defects occur in approximately 1 in 100 babies, many people have heard or read little about them. It is important to remember first that almost all heart defects can now be treated, many in early infancy. Even better, many defects—about one in four—are so mild that they do not need any treatment at all. For practical purposes, the hearts of these infants are normal. As more and more tiny defects in the ventricular septum and minor abnormalities of the heart valves are recognized early in life, the number of children who have defects that need no medical or surgical treatment will continue to rise. Our emphasis in this book is on how such mild defects can be distinguished from severe ones, and what treatments are available when they are needed.

Severe defects require treatment immediately after the child is born. About one in four heart defects is serious enough to need treatment during infancy. Others, less critical—about one-quarter to one-half of all defects—may require treatment as the child grows. Almost all defects can be successfully treated.

Grouping of Congenital Heart Defects

An understanding of how the normal heart develops (see chapter 2) will help in trying to visualize where defects can occur, and how they might be grouped together. The method of grouping or classification used in this book is based on our understanding of how the human heart forms (figure 4.1).

Because the heart starts to function long before birth, its growth and development can be changed by several processes in the womb. There can be disturbances in blood flow into any of the heart chambers. (Disturbed flow may interfere with the normal separation and development of the heart into its four chambers or may contribute to defective growth of the heart valves.) There can be a failure of cells from the primitive nervous system to move normally into the outflow area between the right ventricle and the lungs. (Conotruncal defects are the result of failure of normal movement or migration of specialized cells known as neural crest cells.)

If some of the heart tissue of the early embryo is too sticky or carries abnormal genetic programming, an endocardial cushion (atrioventricular canal) defect results, affecting the tricuspid mitral valves and the septum in the middle of the heart, sometimes called the atrioventricular septum.

About 90 percent of all congenital heart defects result from flow disturbances or conotruncal or endocardial cushion defects (figure 4.2).

Frequency of Groups of Defects

If your own child's heart has a particular defect, such as a ventricular septal defect, do you really care how many other children have a similar one? You probably do. Most parents find it reassuring to know that their child is not alone and that a great deal of knowledge is available on the good outcome of such defects.

Although there are variations among studies, the differences they report are rather minor if one compares the findings in young infants in various parts of the world. Age at the time of study obviously makes a

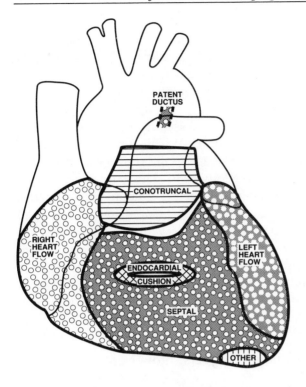

4.1. Grouping of Heart Defects (adapted from a diagram used by Dr. Charlotte Ferencz). **Flow defects** (*bubble pattern*) include (1) atrial and ventricular septal defects and patent ductus, (2) right-heart flow, and (3) left-heart flow defects. **Conotruncal defects** (*horizontal lines*) involve the area of the heart leading from the right ventricle to the lungs. **Endocardial cushion defects** (*cross-hatching*) affect the tricuspid and mitral valves and the central atrioventricular canal area. **Other defects** are rare, and include abnormal looping of the heart and coronary abnormalities.

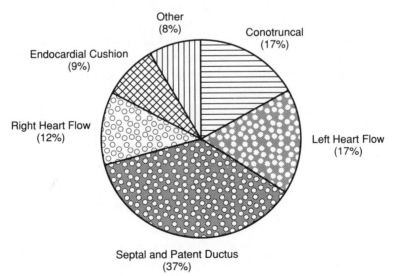

4.2. Incidence of Heart Defects. These figures reflect approximate incidence figures, based in part on the first six years of the Baltimore-Washington Infant Study. Groupings as in figure 4.1.

difference: if a defect is severe, affected children may die in infancy and a study of 5-year-old children would find almost no children with that particular defect. Similarly, mild defects may not be recognized at all in the first year of life and therefore none would be reported in a study of 1-year-olds.

The frequency, or prevalence, figures used here are based on findings in the first six years of the Baltimore-Washington Infant Study. In that study all infants under 1 year of age in the region who had heart defects were registered from 1981 to 1989. This study agrees with many others in showing that septal defects, including patent ductus, are the most common group, accounting for almost four in ten of all heart defects in infants. Because septal defects and patent ductus are among the most easily treated and most benign of all defects, the fact that they are also the most common is gratifying. It means that the overall outlook for children with heart defects is highly positive. (For individual defects, see the table of contents or the index of this book and also chapter cross-references indicated in this chapter.)

The Most Common Defects: Flow Defects

After birth, in atrial septal defects, ventricular septal defects, and patent ductus, the flow of blood is from the left side of the heart to the right (figure 4.3); therefore, too much blood flows into the lungs. The larger the defect, the more the excessive flow into the lungs. These defects are sometimes referred to as "left-to-right shunts," meaning that some blood that should be going to the body is being shunted through the defect and therefore is reaching the lungs instead. Although a persistently patent ductus arteriosus is outside the heart, patent ductus is often included with the left-to-right shunt group of flow defects because it also leads to increased blood flow in the lungs after birth.

Large septal defects and patent ductus can all cause similar problems for a child:

- Rapid breathing even when asleep, a consequence of congested lungs.
- Delayed growth, because extra calories are being used (wasted) by the abnormal circulation and rapid breathing. Usually growth in weight is more delayed than growth in height.
- Sweating, heart failure, and severe difficulty in feeding, which may signal the presence of a large defect that requires early treatment.

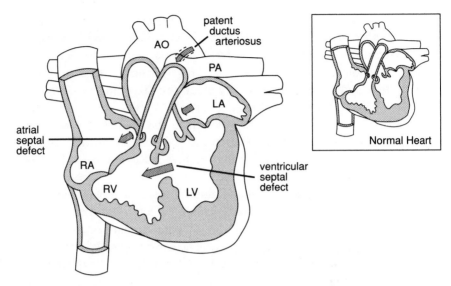

4.3. Flow Defects: Septal Defects and Patent Ductus Arteriosus. The *arrows* show blood flowing from the left side of the heart into the right side in all three types of defect. The ventricular septal defect illustrated is a large one, almost the same size as the opening into the aorta at the aortic valve; such a large defect would almost certainly need surgery. Ninety-five percent of all septal defects are smaller than this one. *Key: AO* = aorta; *PA* = pulmonary artery; *LA* = left atrium; *RA* = right atrium; *RV* = right ventricle; *LV* = left ventricle.

Atrial and Ventricular Septal Defects and Patent Ductus

The walls, or septa, between the right and left sides of the heart are elongated; they develop over a relatively long period of time before birth.

Abnormalities in the development of the walls of the heart or delayed closure of the patent ductus are common, as we have said above, and they are treatable, too, if they are large enough to need any treatment at all—these defects may be so tiny as to be quite insignificant, and may seal off without any treatment. But if there is a large opening or defect in the septum, the consequences can be serious unless heart surgery is performed early in life.

Sometimes people will say of a child with a septal defect that he or she has "a hole in the heart." This colloquial term is accurate—there is, indeed, a hole or perforation in the wall that separates the left from the right side of the heart. The heart is such an important organ that the idea of a hole in it is extremely worrying, of course. Lay people may conjure up pictures of a heart with blood falling out. It is better for the family to know the correct term, and particularly to learn whether the defect is so small that it will need no treatment. The size of the defect is important. These defects vary greatly in size and therefore vary greatly in how severely they may affect the child.

All of these defects are thought to be caused by some abnormality of flow through the heart when the fetus is in the womb. In some cases, genetic factors seem to be the reason for the abnormal flow. In others, no cause can be identified.

In the majority of infants and children, a septal defect or a patent ductus is detected by what is called "**elective referral**"; that is, first a heart murmur is heard, leading the primary-care nurse or physician to seek the advice of a cardiologist. The cardiologist will perform a cardiac evaluation, including an echo-Doppler test, to confirm the presence of a defect and its size.

In other infants a heart murmur may have been present from soon after birth and may have been followed medically without special concern. Then around 2 to 6 months of age the infant contracts a viral illness and, instead of recovering quickly, begins to feed poorly, breathe hard, and sweat excessively while feeding. The pediatrician or family doctor then finds congestion of the lungs and liver and signs of heart failure, and may recommend hospital admission. There, cardiac evaluation with echo-Doppler tests (sometimes followed by cardiac catheterization) leads to confirmation of a large defect, usually a VSD (see below). Rarely does a patent ductus in a full-term infant come to light in this way.

Some infants with heart defects are not in heart failure but are referred for a check for a suspected syndrome, that is, for a collection of abnormalities. For example, in a baby with fetal alcohol syndrome a murmur that is presumed to be caused by a heart defect will be evaluated earlier than would be the case if the baby were otherwise normal.

Atrial septal defects

An ASD is an opening or defect in the middle part of the wall between the right and left atrium. It usually occurs in otherwise healthy children, more often in girls than in boys.

In the womb there is always a small opening in the fetus's atrial septum. Because of its oval shape, this opening is called the foramen ovale (*foramen* = opening). Before birth, blood flows from the right atrium to the left through the foramen. At birth the pressure in the left atrium rises, and blood flow through the foramen ends; eventually the foramen seals off completely. If blood flow into the right ventricle is lower than normal before birth, however, more blood is forced through the atrial septum and a larger than normal opening persists after birth. This is an ASD. Because the pressure is higher in the left atrium than the right after birth, blood flows from the left to the right atrium (arrow in figure 4.3 shows direction of flow through atrial septal defect). As a result of excessive blood flow into the right side of the heart, the right atrium and ventricle and the pulmonary artery all dilate, becoming larger than normal to accommodate the extra blood.

Recognition of atrial septal defects. Most children who have an ASD appear healthy and normally active. Perhaps a child is a little thin, but is able to breathe comfortably. On examination the cardiologist observes a heart murmur. As the child lies quietly on the examining couch for an echo-Doppler test, the doctor can see the movement of the heart through the thin chest wall. The right ventricle may look and feel overactive. On listening with the stethoscope the doctor finds that a second heart sound (the dup-p of the lub dup-p sequence) is abnormal: the two parts of dup-p are wide apart, more like dup—p. The cardiologist can probably tell now, before any further tests are done, whether or not the child has a heart problem such as an ASD.

The echo-Doppler is the "gold standard," even though an ASD can usually be diagnosed with confidence on examination alone. The defect in the wall between the atria can almost always be seen clearly on the echo-Doppler test. Perhaps even more important, it is possible to see that the heart has no other defects. The right atrium and ventricle of the heart are larger than normal for the child's age because of the excess blood flow into them, and the pulmonary artery is also large. Otherwise, the heart is fine and the function of the heart muscle excellent. Additional tests—cardiac catheterization, for example—are very rarely needed.

ASDs vary in the size and position of the defect in the septum. Some defects are extremely small, really just a persistence of the foramen ovale that is normally present in the fetus. Closure of such tiny defects is recommended only rarely. Most ASDs are repaired with surgery in childhood, as described in the story of Janine in the Introduction, and in chapter 12.

Most commonly, the ASD lies in the middle of the septum; a defect higher in the septum is called a sinus venosus defect or, more often, an atrial septal defect with partial anomalous pulmonary venous return. In such cases, one or more of the veins from the right lung connect to the upper part of the right atrium instead of the left atrium, as is normal. A sinus venosus defect is similar to a classical ASD except that the sinus venosus defect is more difficult to see clearly on the echocardiogram, and therefore cardiac catheterization will sometimes be needed before surgery. During surgery a patch is placed inside the atrium to direct the veins back into the left atrium. The patch heals over within three months, leaving a normal, smooth endocardial lining inside the heart. When surgery is performed in adolescence or adulthood, many surgeons recommend the use of anticoagulants for six months after the operation to prevent clot formation on the patch while it is healing. However, clots are so exceptional in young children that this medication is very seldom recommended for them. Abnormal heart rhythms are more frequent with sinus venosus defects than with classical ASDs, both before and after the operation. A sinus venosus defect, like a classical ASD, can be thought of as a heart problem that does need surgical repair but that has an excellent long-term outlook.

A defect low in the atrial septum is sometimes called an **ostium primum**, because it develops earlier in embryonic life than the classical ASD, which is an **ostium secundum**. An ostium primum is a mild form of endocardial cushion defect. Very occasionally, the entire atrial septum is missing, leading to a single atrium, which is also a form of endocardial cushion defect (see chapter 6).

When an ASD exists along with some other problem in the heart, the treatment plan and the timing of surgery depend on the nature and severity of the other defect.

Ventricular septal defects

A ventricular septal defect (VSD) is an opening or defect in the wall or septum between the right and left ventricle (figure 4-3). Most VSDs are in the upper part of the septum, where the septum is thin like a parchment or membrane; they are often called membranous or perimembranous VSDs. It is not surprising they are so frequent, because closure in this area requires at least four different structures to join perfectly together, so there are many possibilities for mistiming. The lower part of the septum is thicker and contains more muscle fibers than the upper membranous part; a defect low in the septum is called a muscular VSD.

Because VSDs are so frequent, you will find many references to them in this book. In this chapter we will summarize how a VSD may affect the child, what the cardiologist may find, and the principles of treatment. The course and treatment of a baby with a VSD depends a great deal on the size of the defect, which can vary from tiny, less than a pinpoint across, to large, almost as big as the opening from the left ventricle into the aorta. Defects of the same size can vary in their effect, depending on whether new findings develop or whether other defects are also present.

As a result of many investigations, including the Natural History Study mentioned earlier, and many more recent studies, including the BWIS, it is now widely agreed that most children born with a VSD grow and develop into healthy adults. In about one child in five the defect closes itself, usually before 2 years of age. Small muscular VSDs have a great tendency to close as the heart muscle grows to keep up with the child's growth. In a majority of children the defect shrinks in size and produces no problem except for a murmur over the heart.

If the defect is large, more than about three millimeters in diameter, many of the symptoms we described earlier can occur; these include rapid breathing, tiring while feeding, sweating, slow weight gain, and a risk that simple colds may lead to chest infections or even pneumonia. A heart murmur is nearly always heard; rarely, when the defect is very large, the murmur may be difficult to hear. Sometimes, as in the story of Andrew in the Introduction and Carlos in chapter 12, symptoms do not come on right after birth, but are delayed for a few weeks. If the cardiologist finds signs of heart failure—such as an engorged liver, a pile-up of fluid in the lungs, and a greatly increased heart rate and rate of breathing—immediate surgery may be recommended, sometimes preceded by a cardiac catheterization test. If no urgent signs are present, a little time may be spent with medical treatment, to allow the defect a chance to get smaller. Almost all large VSDs can now be closed successfully, even in very small babies. Occasionally a very tiny infant, weighing only one or two pounds, may need an operation that can be done quickly and does not involve the heart-lung machine. This operation, known as banding of the pulmonary artery, allows the baby to grow in size and strength and to have the defect repaired at a few months old.

What about the baby who has a defect that is neither small nor large, but somewhere in between? This is often referred to as a "moderate" VSD. A recommendation about surgery will be guided by how well the baby is feeding and growing.

Each baby is different, as all parents know who have had more than one child. So not every baby fits neatly into the scheme of small, moderate, or large VSD outlined here and in other resource books. There can be several variations. Sometimes there are several defects in the muscular part of the septum, which looks riddled with holes and is called a "Swiss cheese" type of septal defect. In other children the aortic valve is involved in the VSD and gradually becomes leaky from constantly being pulled down into the defect with each heartbeat. The child has a VSD with aortic insufficiency. Other babies, about one in thirty of those with large or moderate VSD, develop some pulmonic stenosis as they grow and need surgery for the combination of problems. A VSD may also be seen with other heart defects, such as coarctation of the aorta. Frequently, both defects can be treated at the same operation, but occasionally it is best to treat in stages.

Before surgery could be done in infancy, some babies with large VSDs developed very high pressure in the lungs, so that blood eventually flowed from the right to the left ventricle, and the child became blue (cyanotic). This complication, the Eisenmenger reaction or Eisenmenger syndrome, is now, fortunately, almost never seen.

Later in the book we will describe the stories of some children with different types of VSD. Overall, these children do very well, as most defects get smaller and those that remain large can be repaired early in life. We now anticipate that babies who are born without additional major problems inside or outside the heart have a 90 to 95 percent chance of having a normal adult life.

Patent ductus arteriosus

Patent ductus arteriosus (see figure 4.3) is a persistence after birth of the fetal channel or ductus that has joined the aorta and the pulmonary artery. In the fetus, blood flows from the pulmonary artery to the aorta down the ductus, but at birth the muscle in the wall of the ductus normally tightens up or constricts because it is sensitive to the new, higher level of oxygen in the blood. Blood thus stops passing through the ductus a few hours after birth. However, the ductus may remain open after birth, either in a small premature infant whose ductus muscle is not mature enough to react to changes in oxygen (the most usual case) or, much less frequently, in a full-term infant whose ductus muscle is defective.

Immediately after birth, blood flow through the ductus is usually from the aorta to the pulmonary artery because the pressure in the aorta is now higher. Only if there is a severe lung problem does blood flow from the right side of the heart to the left side, as it did before birth.

Occasionally, all three types of defect occur together, and the child has an open (patent) ductus and both an ASD and a VSD. Fortunately, all three of these defects can usually be repaired in surgery at the same time.

Patent ductus arteriosus was once one of the most common defects occurring in the heart, but now, if we exclude premature babies (especially those under one thousand grams), patent ductus is quite rare, probably because mothers no longer have rubella (German measles) during pregnancy since the availability of vaccine. Occasionally patent ductus runs in a family; in one family, the mother and her twin daughters all had this problem. The mother was an adult before she knew she had a defect, and she has remained so healthy that she has always refused an operation to repair it. In both her daughters, however, the patent ductus was closed surgically. There are now three healthy grandchildren, all with normal hearts.

Usually a patent ductus is detected in a baby or young child because the physician hears a heart murmur characteristic of this defect. Unless there are other signs or symptoms, such as heart failure, most cardiologists will advise waiting until the baby is 1 year old before operating, to allow time for the duct to close itself if it will. Surgery can be done, if the baby is full-term and not in heart failure, at any age; it is usually performed when the child is between 1 and 2 years of age.

Medications to keep the ductus arteriosus open or to close it can be important in the newborn's first days or weeks. The ductus, an artery joining the aorta and the pulmonary artery that is important in the circulation before birth, closes shortly after the baby with a normal ductus is born. Administration of indomethacin to a premature baby whose ductus has failed to close properly will make the ductus close, thus avoiding the need for surgery.

Surgery will prevent the heart from enlarging later and also will prevent bacterial endocarditis, an infection that used to be particularly common with this defect (see chapter 14). Surgery has been done successfully since 1939, so we have had fifty years of experience in followup. A number of people who have had this operation later served in the armed forces or excelled in athletics. In some newborn babies with severe heart defects it may be valuable to keep the ductus *open* for a time after birth with a medication called prostaglandin E1 (see chapter 10).

Valves of the Heart

In infants in whom septation (the division of the heart into two sides) is normal, the valves or the chambers on one side or the other may fail to develop properly, probably because blood flow through the heart has been disturbed in some way before birth. Usually such obstruction is caused by thickening of one or more of the heart valves: if the valve leading into or out of a ventricle is badly malformed, the ventricle itself may fail to grow and at birth may be too small to take over its role as an effective pumping chamber. When the tricuspid or pulmonary valve, the pulmonary artery, or the right ventricle is abnormal, we say that a right-heart flow defect is present. Such defects range from a mild bicuspid pulmonary valve to the severe problem of a hypoplastic (small) right ventricle, which requires treatment immediately after birth. When the obstruction involves the left side of the heart, the mitral or aortic valve, or the aorta or the left ventricle, a left-heart flow defect is present. These defects also vary a great deal in severity, from a mild bicuspid aortic valve to the life-threatening hypoplastic left ventricle. (These defects, like the others noted before, are discussed in more detail in the chapters that follow.)

Right-heart flow defects

In a child with a right-heart flow defect there is an obstacle to the normal, smooth flow of blood from the right side of the heart into the lungs (figure 4.4). These defects range from the very mild, requiring no treatment at all, to the very severe, requiring one or more of many different procedures and operations. Defects at the far end of the spectrum of severity, such as **pulmonary atresia** (atresia = failure of development) with a hypoplastic right ventricle, can have serious consequences; those closer to the middle of the spectrum are milder and more readily treatable.

Bicuspid pulmonary valve. In the very mildest form of right-heart flow problems, the pulmonary valve has only two cusps (leaflets) instead of the normal three. A bicuspid pulmonary valve is really just a very minor variation on the normal valve, a bit like having a web between the third and fourth toes—a little unusual, but of no consequence. In fact, the only sign of such a trivial variation is a faint clicking sound made by the valve as it opens; the sound may be heard when the child's heart is being examined and may lead the doctor to recommend an echocar-

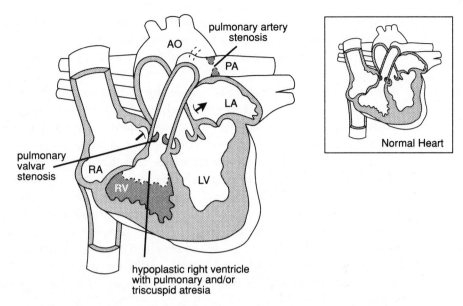

4.4. Right-Heart Flow Defects. In *pulmonary arterial stenosis* there is narrowing of one or both pulmonary arteries. In *pulmonary valvar stenosis*, the leaflets of the pulmonary valve are thickened; the valve does not open fully with each heartbeat. In *hypoplastic right ventricle* the cavity of the right ventricle is small (*dark shading*); either the pulmonary or tricuspid valve (or both) are sealed closed or atretic. Often blood passes from the right atrium to the left (*arrow*) because it has no outlet from the tiny, thick-walled right ventricle.

diogram to confirm that there are only two cusps to the valve. If everything else in the heart is normal, there is no need for any treatment or follow-up visits to a cardiologist.

Pulmonary valve stenosis. In other children the leaflets of the pulmonary valve are thickened and not separated from each other, but partially tethered together, resulting in some narrowing (stenosis) of the valve, so that it does not open up as widely as normal with each heartbeat. Pulmonary valve stenosis is the most frequent right-heart flow defect; it was found in about 8 of 100 children with heart defects in the large Ontario Heart Registry and in 7 of 100 infants registered in the BWIS. In almost all children with pulmonary valve stenosis the first indication is a heart murmur, usually heard quite early in infancy, which gradually becomes a little louder.

Very occasionally the pulmonary valve is so narrow that it produces symptoms immediately after birth. Blood has difficulty passing through the narrow valve into the lungs and instead backs up in the veins in the body; as a result, the liver becomes enlarged, and sometimes fluid gathers in the body tissues and around the eyes, producing **edema**. All these findings indicate heart failure and require emergency treatment.

When a stenotic (narrowed) valve opens it does not open completely, but instead the tethered leaflets dome upward together. Sometimes the opening in the valve is very narrow—usually one-half or two-thirds the normal size—and blood has great difficulty getting through to the lungs. As blood forces its way through the narrowed valve, a click and loud heart murmur are produced. The right ventricle has to pump harder than normal, and at a higher pressure, to force blood through the narrowed valve. The normal pressure in the right ventricle when the pulmonary valve opens is between 20 and 25 mm Hg, about one-fifth that in the left ventricle. The right ventricle tolerates a pressure of 40 to 50 mm Hg well, but higher pressures may lead to thickening of the muscle wall and gradual failure of the heart muscle (see figure 1.5).

Dysplastic pulmonary valve. In about 5 of 100 children with pulmonary stenosis the valve is thick and knobby and does not open up well with the balloon catheter. This type of dysplastic pulmonary valve is rare in children who are otherwise normal, but it is often seen as part of a syndrome of slow growth called Noonan-Ehmke syndrome (see chapter 15).

Peripheral pulmonary stenosis. In peripheral pulmonary stenosis the narrowing is beyond the valve, in the wall of one or both pulmonary arteries. Such narrowing, unusual by itself, is more often seen in children with tetralogy of Fallot or with other heart disorders involving abnormal growth of the pulmonary arteries. When peripheral pulmonary stenosis is the only defect, it is usually quite mild and its only effect is to cause a heart murmur. Treatment is hardly ever necessary, and the child can lead a normal life.

Infundibular pulmonary stenosis. Pulmonary stenosis occurs below the valve, rather than at the valve itself, in 1 in 300 children who have pulmonary stenosis without any other defect in the heart. This narrowing below the valve is called "infundibular pulmonary stenosis" and usually requires surgery.

Hypoplastic right ventricle (with atresia of the pulmonary or tricuspid valve). For a child with a hypoplastic right ventricle, the health team and the family have many hurdles to cross and many hard decisions to make in trying to restore the child's heart to a near-healthy state. In this condition the ventricle is a tiny muscle-bound slit instead of the efficient pumping chamber of the healthy newborn heart. This is a very serious condition.

Hypoplastic right ventricle in the newborn is a cardiac emergency because there is

- Too little blood flow to the lungs, which in turn causes
- Too little oxygen in the blood, which leads to
- Intense cyanosis or blueness that does not improve with administration of oxygen.

While the infant is still in the womb there is no sign of difficulty. Growth tends to be a little slow, and the baby's birth weight is often in the low-normal range. Oxygen is being supplied by the placenta, so all of the other organs develop normally. But almost immediately after birth the infant is blue (cyanotic). Often this cyanosis is very severe and does not respond at all to treatment with an oxygen hood. This intense blueness, combined with a heart murmur and an abnormal chest X-ray and electrocardiogram, usually leads to urgent cardiac referral within the first day or two of life. Often the baby is started on an intravenous course of prostaglandin to keep the ductus open, while plans are being developed for the baby's transfer and treatment (see chapter 10).

If you look at figure 4.4 you can see that when the right ventricle is small (shown diagrammatically as dark shading), the blood flow to the lungs will be much reduced. Sometimes the pulmonary valve, instead of being stenotic or narrow, is completely closed. In this condition of pulmonary atresia the right ventricle is a thick-walled blind cavity, and all blood flow to the lungs depends entirely on the ductus. If the ductus is allowed to close, the baby cannot survive.

In other babies with **tricuspid atresia**, the tricuspid valve may have failed to form and at birth is sealed shut. Sometimes there is a small ventricular septal defect, allowing some blood to reach the right ventricle and pulmonary artery, but the amount of blood reaching the lungs is severely reduced. Any baby with a hypoplastic right ventricle needs urgent treatment in the newborn period and may need more than one operation (see chapter 10).

Left-heart flow defects

In a child with a left-heart flow defect there is an obstacle to the normal, smooth flow of blood from the left side of the heart to the aorta and the body (figure 4.5). Such defects range in severity from very mild defects that need little if any treatment, such as bicuspid aortic valve, to the most severe and life-threatening defects, such as hypoplastic left ventricle.

Bicuspid aortic valve. In the mildest type of left-heart flow defect, the aortic valve has only two leaflets or cusps instead of the normal three. Such a bicuspid aortic valve does not give rise to any difficulty in childhood. Indeed, it is so mild that there is a great discrepancy between the number of times it is diagnosed and its true frequency. Probably as many as 1 in 100 people have two rather than three cusps, but very few of them are aware of it. In childhood the only sign is a clicking sound, often not very loud, heard as the valve opens. An echo-Doppler test can confirm whether the valve has the usual number of cusps. Does it matter? It does matter, because although the bicuspid aortic valve functions well, it lacks the perfect engineering design of the three-leaflet valve, and problems may develop later.

A bicuspid aortic valve may lead to three types of problems. First, the valve is more likely to become infected from bacteria in the bloodstream—endocarditis is a risk, although a low one, and these children need BE prophylaxis (see chapter 14) before surgical or dental procedures. Second, the valve may become leaky during the teenage years, so a checkup at between 10 and 15 years of age is advisable. Third, in middle age the valve may become thickened by calcium deposits, becoming narrow enough to need surgical replacement. Bicuspid aortic valve is a kind of "sleeper" defect; it is almost never a problem in childhood, but it may cause trouble many years later.

Aortic valve stenosis. If the normally delicate leaflets of the aortic valve are tethered together and thickened, the opening in the valve may be narrowed or stenotic and obstruct the normal, easy flow of blood from the left ventricle to the aorta. In aortic valve stenosis the valve leaflets do not open completely with each heartbeat. The stenosis may be severe, requiring emergency treatment in infancy. More often it becomes gradually more severe with growth, requiring treatment at some time during childhood (see chapter 12).

In the past, a child with a heart murmur and a click (the sound of

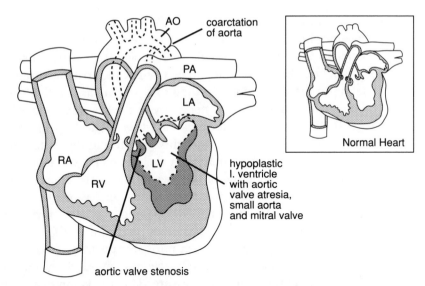

4.5. Left-Heart Flow Defects. In *coarctation* the aorta (*AO*) is narrowed close to where the ductus (shown as *two dotted lines*) joins the pulmonary artery (*PA*) and aorta. This results in obstruction of blood flow to the lower part of the body. In *aortic valve stenosis* the aortic valve leaflets are thickened and the valve does not open fully with each heartbeat. In *hypoplastic left ventricle* the cavity of the left ventricle (*LV*) is small (*dark shading*) and the aorta is tiny; either the aortic or mitral valve or both are sealed closed or atretic. Blood flow to the body after birth comes from the right ventricle (*RV*) and can continue only while the ductus remains open.

an opening heart valve) who was completely free of symptoms might not be referred to a cardiologist until he or she was 5 years old and ready to start school. It often came as a great shock to the family at that time to learn that the child had a narrow valve that might need surgery. Nowadays, such children are usually referred to a cardiologist early on; the family can see the valve on the echo tape and discuss with the cardiologist how severe the narrowing is and whether and how often follow-up will be necessary.

In earlier years, a condition such as aortic valve stenosis—which is more frequent in boys than in girls—presented a great problem, especially for children eager to go out for sports; it was known that the narrowing of the valve became more severe over time, but there was no good way of monitoring the change other than by repeated catheter tests. Now the severity of the narrowing can be accurately assessed with the echo-Doppler, and if it is not severe, unnecessary restrictions on a child's activity can be avoided. Occasionally, in about one in twenty children who have aortic valve stenosis, the valve is severely narrowed and badly formed. Such a baby will have a heart murmur, will be breathing fast, and will be restless and irritable; fluid is accumulating in the lungs, often leading to wheezing and difficulty in feeding. Emergency surgery will be necessary in the first days or weeks of life.

If the aortic valve is thickened there is a drop in pressure, also called a **gradient**, between the left ventricle and the aorta. This gradient can be measured accurately with the Doppler test; such measurement allows an understanding of how severe the obstruction is and provides a way of monitoring its progression over time. When the aortic valve is greatly thickened, with a narrow opening, the left ventricular pressure may be between 150 and 200 when pressure in the aorta is around 100. Maintaining a higher than normal pressure is a strain on the left ventricle. The muscle of the ventricle, the myocardium, thickens in order to maintain the needed pressure. This thickening (hypertrophy) is well tolerated if it is mild, but if the myocardium becomes greatly thickened, the blood supply from the coronary arteries to the muscle becomes inadequate, particularly during strenuous exercise. In general, a cardiologist will follow a child with aortic valve stenosis and recommend treatment if the pressure is 1.5 times greater (or more) in the left ventricle than in the aorta (for example, 150 mm Hg in the ventricle, 100 mm Hg in the aorta).

The child with aortic valve stenosis will not need any medication other than BE prophylaxis but will usually need to be checked annually during the childhood years of rapid growth to make sure that the opening in the valve is growing and keeping up with the needs of the growing body.

Coarctation of the aorta. Coarctation is a narrowing of the aorta, causing obstruction of a smooth flow of blood from the upper to the lower part of the body. It leads to higher blood pressure in the arms than in the legs. The problem lies in the aorta beyond the aortic arch, in the area where the ductus arteriosus joins the aorta with the pulmonary artery (figure 4.5). During early development, blood flowing from the pulmonary artery toward the aorta branches; most of the blood flows down to the abdomen and lower limbs but some flows upward toward the head. If some factor reduces flow in the aorta during development, the branch-point of the aorta is narrowed where the ductus joins it. Most of the time the narrowing is a localized shelf, but in some severe variants the aortic arch is narrowed for most of its length. Coarctation can be present with or without aortic valve stenosis.

How does this coarctation come about? During life in the mother's womb the local narrowing of the aorta causes no difficulty, since extra blood needed by the body is pumped from the right ventricle down the ductus, essentially bypassing the narrow area. In many babies the ductus remains open for several days after birth and the circulation continues much as before. However, once the ductus closes, two things happen: first, the ductus shortens to a thin cord, pulling on the coarctation shelf area and making it narrower; second, the left ventricle now has to pump blood directly through the obstruction, since the bypass down the duct no longer exists, and the left ventricle often fails as a result. These events lead to a sudden change from a healthy baby to one who is breathing hard, sweating, and sometimes even wheezing from accumulation of fluid in the lungs. This sudden change leads to cardiac evaluation as an emergency (see chapter 10).

Coarctation may be recognized in infancy either because of the sudden onset of heart failure between 1 week and 3 months of age or because of a finding of a higher blood pressure and a stronger pulse in the arms than in the legs.

Heart murmurs, often so helpful in directing attention to the heart, are rather insignificant in many babies with coarctation. However, almost half of these infants have, in addition, a bicuspid aortic valve, and many times a click and faint murmur may be noticed coming from this valve. In other infants with coarctation, perhaps as many as one in four, there is also a VSD, which produces a loud murmur. Coarctation can be recognized in these four very different ways:

- Heart failure may suddenly develop in early infancy, usually before 6 weeks of age, as the ductus closes.
- On examination, the pulse may be found stronger and the blood pressure higher in the arms than in the legs.
- The raised blood pressure in the arms may lead to referral for treatment of hypertension and the diagnosis can be made then, sometimes even as late as adulthood.
- A heart murmur from an additional heart defect, such as a VSD, may lead to cardiac evaluation and detection of a coarctation.

A baby who is in heart failure from coarctation may already have been started on prostaglandin treatment before being transferred from the newborn nursery to the cardiac center. If medical treatment has successfully reopened the ductus the signs of heart failure will have lessened and often the difference between arm and leg blood pressures has become less pronounced than earlier. However, some difference persists. The narrowing of the aorta can be seen on an echocardiogram, and the Doppler test will confirm a drop in pressure across the coarctation. A cardiac catheter test may be advised, but echo-Doppler tests are improving and the anatomy can often be seen well enough on this test to preclude the need for any further studies.

In other children the ductus closes off more slowly, and heart failure never develops. These children may appear quite healthy. However, the blood pressure in the arms, above the coarctation, is higher than that in the legs. This difference in pulse and blood pressure is observed on physical examination and leads to a cardiac referral. Even today a child with a coarctation may appear so healthy that no problem is recognized until the teens, when a higher than normal blood pressure in the arms leads to the diagnosis.

The presence of additional defects with coarctation may make early treatment and control more difficult. When a VSD is also present, it is usually not large, and it generally gets smaller or closes as the child grows. When the VSD is large, however, individual planning is needed for the best way to proceed. Quite often the coarctation is repaired first and the baby is kept on medication for a few weeks in the hope that the VSD will decrease in size; if it does not, the VSD is closed in surgery. In extremely sick infants it is now possible to repair both defects at once.

Coarctation is sometimes part of an immensely complex heart defect. For example, a baby may have a single ventricle or some other severe heart problem in addition to coarctation. In such a baby repairing the narrowing in the aorta is but the first step in what may be a long and difficult series of operations and interventions. Fortunately, fewer than one infant in ten who has coarctation has an additional complex heart problem.

In **interrupted aortic arch**, when coarctation is so severe as to result in complete separation of the upper and lower aorta, a large VSD is nearly always also present. Babies with this severe defect become acutely ill a few days after birth, as the ductus begins to close. Treatment with prostaglandins will keep the ductus open until surgery to close the VSD and to bring together the two separated ends of the aorta. This procedure requires a skillful surgeon and use of the heart-lung machine. Interrupted aortic arch is one of the many heart problems now often successfully managed that were always fatal a few short years ago. Babies with interrupted aortic arch often have such problems outside the heart as, for example, Di George syndrome, with low calcium levels in the blood and other difficulties (see chapter 15).

Hypoplastic left ventricle (with atresia of the aortic or mitral valve). Until very recently, infants with a hypoplastic left ventricle always died before 3 months of age, usually in the first week of life. Since 1983 treatment has been possible, although only a few cardiac centers have had any consistent success with surgery. The correct approach remains a subject of debate, and making a decision places great stress on the family and the health team. Hypoplastic left ventricle (also called hypoplastic left heart syndrome) remains a severe heart defect (see chapter 10).

The fundamental problem in hypoplastic left ventricle is failure of development of the left ventricle. If you place your hand on the most forceful part of your own heartbeat, just under the left nipple, you will feel your own left ventricle beating. It is this ventricle that pumps blood to the body, brain, kidneys, and all other organs except the lungs. The pulse in the wrist is propelled there by the force of the beating left ventricle. The left ventricle is the master of the circulation.

When the left ventricle fails to develop, the circulation is extremely abnormal. Both before and after birth, the right ventricle is called upon to do all the work. Blood goes from the right ventricle to the pulmonary artery and from there down the ductus; some blood goes back up the aorta to the head and even back to the aortic valve to supply the coronary arteries. When aortic atresia is present, as it is in most infants who have a hypoplastic left ventricle, the aortic valve is completely closed, so the only blood reaching the heart muscle through the coronary arteries has to come from the right ventricle. Mitral valve atresia also causes the left ventricle to be small, and the baby has the same problems found with aortic atresia. In mitral valve atresia the two leaflets of the mitral valve are stuck together, or atretic, and cannot open to allow blood to flow from the left atrium into the left ventricle.

Everything depends on the ductus; as long as it is open, life can continue, even though the course of the circulation is bizarre. But once the ductus starts to close, no blood can reach the body. There are variations in the size of the left ventricle, which may resemble a withered walnut with almost no cavity or may be a little nearer to normal size. The aortic valve may not be completely sealed shut. There are other variations in defects, including the severity of aortic coarctation. Each infant is affected slightly differently. The child's cardiologist will review with the parents the details of the problem and the treatment. The basic problem is the hypoplastic (small) left ventricle, which has resulted in a circulation entirely dependent on flow through the ductus.

When the left ventricle fails to grow normally, the right ventricle is able to keep the circulation going during life in the womb; the fetus grows a little slowly, but usually there is no difficulty before birth. Sometimes the problem has been recognized in advance by means of fetal echocardiography, and special follow-up has been arranged so that the infant can be delivered in a center with facilities for treatment immediately after birth. Most often, however, a baby is born with no one suspecting that a serious defect of this sort is present. At birth the ductus remains open and the baby may appear normal for a few hours or even a few days. As soon as the ductus starts to close the pulse becomes weak, the baby appears pale and has a mottled color, and a heart murmur may develop.

The sudden collapse of a previously healthy baby is a difficult challenge even if it occurs while the baby is still in the newborn nursery at the hospital. Sometimes the infant is already home before signs develop. If the medication prostaglandin E1 is started quickly, the ductus will reopen and there will be time to consider the various options for treatment. Without prostaglandins, death usually ensues within a few hours or days.

In most babies a severe problem is suspected in the nursery because doctors find a weak pulse and an overactive right ventricle. Cardiac studies are then done, including chest X-ray, electrocardiogram, and Doppler-echocardiogram. Prostaglandins are started and the baby is transferred to a cardiac center.

Usually, by the time prostaglandins have been given for a few hours, the baby's color is back to normal and the cardiologist is able to do a detailed echo-Doppler study to define exactly the size of the left ventricle and the nature of the other problems in the heart.

Sometimes the closure of the ductus is very sudden, and even after prostaglandins are started the blood pressure never becomes normal. The baby remains pale and mottled and blood studies show that the entire metabolism or chemistry of the body has become faulty. **Acidosis** exists; the delicate balance of acids and base substances in the blood has broken down because blood is not reaching the tissues under nor-

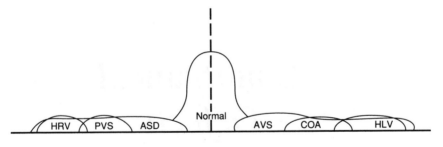

Decreasing Right Heart Flow ◀ ▶ **Decreasing Left Heart Flow**

4.6. Flow Defects: The Spectrum of Severity. *Key: HRV* = hypoplastic right ventricle; *PVS* = pulmonary valve stenosis; *ASD* = atrial septal defect; *AVS* = aortic valve stenosis; *COA* = coarctation of aorta; *HLV* = hypoplastic left ventricle.

mal pressure. The outlook for this baby is bleak unless the acidosis can be quickly reversed after prostaglandins are started.

In these infants, as in those with any heart defect, other abnormalities may be present. Approximately 10 percent of babies who have a hypoplastic left ventricle, for example, have a major chromosomal disorder, and another 15 percent may have defects of the central nervous system or other organs. In almost 75 percent of babies, however, the heart defect is the only problem.

Developmental defects caused by abnormal flow through the heart while the baby is in the womb are important because they are so common. They vary a great deal in how they affect the child after birth, but almost all can now be successfully treated with a combination of medications and surgery. Figure 4.6 shows diagrammatically how right- and left-heart flow defects form a spectrum from the mildest to the most severe. Recent advances in medical and surgical treatment are providing increasing hope even for infants with hypoplastic right or left ventricles, who are at the extremes of the spectrum of severity.

Chapter 5

Conotruncal Defects

In the normal heart, blood returning from the body passes to the right ventricle, the pulmonary artery, and then to the lungs to receive a new supply of oxygen. The conotruncal area of the heart provides this vital connection between heart and lungs. When this area has not developed normally before birth, blood does not reach the lungs as it should and oxygen levels in the blood are too low. This low oxygen level in the arteries and tissues of the body results in a blue color known as cyanosis, from the Greek word *cyan* (blue).

The skin of newborn babies often shows a bluish color immediately after birth, but after a few vigorous cries the lungs fill with oxygen and the blueness disappears. A baby who remains persistently blue, even after the administration of oxygen, is said to be cyanotic. Cyanosis is sometimes caused by a problem in the lungs requiring treatment with a ventilator. In other infants cyanosis is due to a conotruncal heart defect, usually either tetralogy of Fallot or transposition of the great arteries. All conotruncal defects are serious and require surgery, which can now usually be performed in the first weeks or months of life.

Tetralogy of Fallot

Tetralogy of Fallot (named for the nineteenth-century French cardiologist Arthur Fallot) is the most usual cause of cardiac cyanosis, occurring in about three of every ten thousand children born. Successful treatment first became available more than forty years ago; a number of adults who are now leading healthy lives were born with this defect and had successful surgery.

The word *tetralogy* (from the Greek *tetra*, four) implies correctly that there are four defects. Two of these are of major importance. The first, *pulmonary stenosis*, is an obstruction of blood flow to the lungs resulting from a narrowing of the outflow area connecting the right ventricle to the pulmonary artery. It usually affects the pulmonary valve and the infundibular area below the valve. The more severe the pulmonary stenosis, the less blood reaches the child's lungs with each heartbeat, and the worse the cyanosis or blueness. The second important defect is a large ventricular septal defect, causing blood to mix freely between the two ventricles (figure 5.1).

In addition to the two major defects, tetralogy includes two minor, or secondary, defects. The first is an *overriding aorta*. The term *overriding* means that the ventricular septal defect lies immediately beneath the aorta, so the aorta "overrides" both the right and the left ventricle. The aorta receives blue venous blood from the right ventricle mixed with normal, fully oxygenated blood from the left ventricle, a mix that results in cyanosis. The other minor defect is thickening of the right ventricular wall, or *right ventricular hypertrophy*, which develops when the ventricular septal defect is large and causes equal pressure in the right and left ventricles; the wall of the right ventricle then becomes thickened or hypertrophied as a result of this high pressure.

Variants of tetralogy of Fallot are important, because they may affect the timing of surgical repair and how much can be accomplished in one operation.

Tetralogy with pulmonary atresia

The most frequent and important variant, tetralogy with pulmonary atresia, occurred in one in five infants with tetralogy who were in the Baltimore-Washington Infant Study. This condition is much more difficult to treat than the more usual tetralogy, which includes pulmonary stenosis. Also, babies with this condition are at higher risk for problems other than problems of the heart and are often of low birth weight.

With pulmonary atresia there is a complete blockage or obstruction to blood flow into the lungs, and the infant is intensely blue immediately after birth. Sometimes the pulmonary valve is completely closed, and sometimes the pulmonary artery is missing or replaced by a thin cord of fibrous tissue through which no blood can pass. This condition

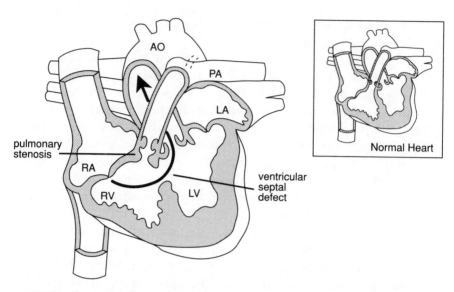

5.1. Tetralogy of Fallot. Pulmonary stenosis is present below the pulmonary valve, so blood flow from the right ventricle (*RV*) to the pulmonary artery (*PA*) is obstructed. Blue venous blood is shown with the *arrow* to pass from the right ventricle through the large ventricular septal defect into the aorta (*AO*). Because the aorta is connected to both ventricles, it is said to be overriding. The wall of the right ventricle is thickened (right ventricular hypertrophy).

nearly always requires more than one operation. Despite all the problems along the way—and there are many—the majority of these babies can be helped.

Tetralogy with absent pulmonary valve

This variant has a somewhat misleading name, since the valve is not completely missing; rather, instead of the normal delicate pulmonary valve leaflets there are only little nodules. The valve is unable to close, and, even during life in the womb, blood leaks back and forth between the pulmonary artery and the right ventricle. The pulmonary artery enlarges, pressing on the bronchi and causing severe breathing difficulty after birth. The principal problem for the infant is not cyanosis but breathing difficulty and lung infections. In other children either the right or left branch of the pulmonary artery may be absent, or other parts of the heart may be defective. All such variants make early successful repair more difficult; more than one operation may be needed. Increasingly, as in babies born with formerly untreatable variants of tetralogy, surgery and special "interventional catheterization" procedures are used together at different stages to make the heart and lung circulation as close to normal as possible.

Tetralogy was first treated surgically in 1944, when Drs. Blalock and Taussig succeeded in improving the lack of oxygen in the blood by creating the Blalock-Taussig shunt (see the Introduction). This was a closed-heart operation, meaning that the heart-lung machine was not used; the operation involved arteries in the chest but outside the heart itself. This operation is still useful for a number of babies. (See figure 13.1.) More and more often, however, a single operation called "open repair," using the heart-lung machine, is done when the baby is a few months old; the ventricular septal defect is repaired and the obstructing pulmonary stenosis is removed. Increasingly, therefore, a baby born with tetralogy will reach the first birthday no longer blue or cyanotic, but growing well and acting like a perfectly healthy child. Later in the book we will tell the stories of some infants who were born with tetralogy. In chapter 12 we provide more details of surgical treatment and discuss what the families of these infants can expect after the operation.

Transposition

Transposition is also referred to as transposition of the great arteries and sometimes, as d-transposition (*d* is short for the Latin *dextro*, right), a medical shorthand term meaning that the aorta is transposed from its normal position and lies to the right of the pulmonary artery. (In *levo*- or *l*-transposition, the aorta is connected to the right ventricle but lies to the left of the pulmonary artery; this is a rare condition not discussed in this book.)

In transposition the great arteries are wrongly connected with the heart. The aorta connects to the right ventricle (receiving blue venous blood from it) instead of to the left. The pulmonary artery is connected to the left ventricle, which receives red blood full of oxygen (figure 5.2). Venous blood returning to the heart passes normally into the right ventricle but then is routed back to the aorta. In transposition, blood coming back from the body does not reach the lungs for a fresh supply of oxygen.

Transposition is a serious defect of the heart, but it has seen a more dramatic change in outlook than any other single heart problem. Until the mid-1960s infants with transposition died from complications of

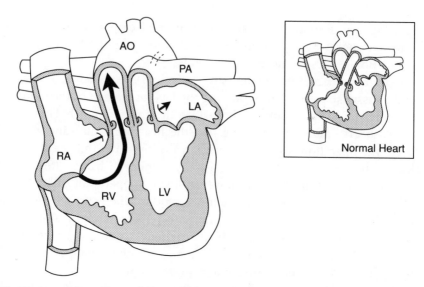

Normal Heart

5.2. Transposition. The arteries are wrongly connected to the heart, or transposed. The *large arrow* shows blue venous blood going from the right ventricle (*RV*) to the aorta (*AO*). Blood from the lungs comes back to the left atrium (*LA*), left ventricle (*LV*), and back via the pulmonary artery (*PA*) to the lungs. The two circulations connect only by temporary openings, the foramen ovale in the atrial septum (*small arrow*), and the ductus (*dotted lines* connecting aorta and pulmonary artery).

low blood oxygen (**hypoxia**) before their first birthday. It is now possible for some such infants to receive successful correction of transposition in the first few days of life. They go home a healthy pink color and with their great arteries no longer transposed (see chapter 10).

Other Conotruncal Defects

Rarer defects in the conotruncal area of the heart include double outlet right ventricle, truncus arteriosus, and aortopulmonary window.

Double outlet right ventricle

In double outlet right ventricle both the aorta and the pulmonary artery arise from the right ventricle; a large ventricular septal defect is usually also present (figure 5.3). Some of these babies have severe pulmonary stenosis and are intensely blue. Many of them can eventually have successful surgery, but usually more than one operation is needed.

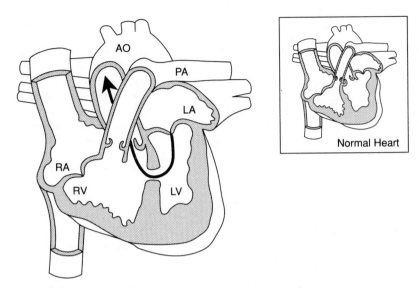

5.3. Double Outlet Right Ventricle. Both the aorta (*AO*) and pulmonary artery (*PA*) arise from the right ventricle (*RV*). The left ventricle (*LV*) has no artery leaving it. The only exit from the *LV* is through a defect in the ventricular septum, shown with *arrow*.

Additional defects outside the heart are common in such cases, so this remains a challenging and difficult type of heart defect. When there is no pulmonary stenosis the baby often does not appear blue but is in heart failure. It is sometimes possible to correct the defect in a one-stage operation, but often in such cases two procedures are needed.

Truncus arteriosus

Truncus arteriosus is a rare condition in which the aorta and pulmonary artery have failed to separate and remain joined as one big artery leaving the heart, overriding a large ventricular septal defect (figure 5.4). Successful surgery to separate the two vessels is now possible in early infancy. The surgery is difficult and often requires the use of an artificial valve. These children need careful follow-up even after successful surgery. Infants born with truncus arteriosus often have a poorly developed thymus gland and other features of Di George syndrome (a condition with a cluster of defects), which may complicate their course before and after surgery.

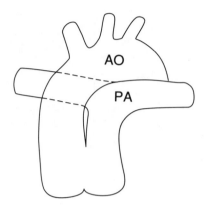

5.4. Truncus Arteriosus. The aorta (*AO*) and pulmonary artery (*PA*) have failed to separate. There is a single valve on the truncus. A large ventricular septal defect is always present (not shown). The pulmonary arteries may arise together or separately from the truncus. In either case surgery is needed in early infancy.

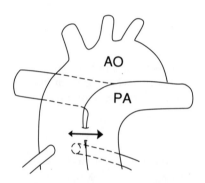

5.5. Aortopulmonary Window. An aortopulmonary window is an opening between the aorta (*AO*) and pulmonary artery (*PA*) a little after they leave the heart. It is a rare defect that can be repaired in infancy using cardiopulmonary bypass.

Aortopulmonary window

Aortopulmonary window, a rare condition, is rather like a truncus, but less severe. In this condition there are separate aortic and pulmonary valves (figure 5.5). The defect is between the aorta and the pulmonary artery a little after they leave the heart. Defects outside the heart are unusual in children with aortopulmonary window, and surgery (requiring a heart-lung machine) is usually quite successful.

Further advances in fetal echocardiography will help us identify the early stages of conotruncal defects during the mother's pregnancy, and eventually, perhaps, we will be able to treat them before birth. Most important of all, as we learn more about the interactions between the developing heart and the nervous system, we will learn why some children are born with multiple handicaps, and how these tragedies can be avoided.

Chapter 6

Endocardial Cushion
Defects

Early in the development of the fetal heart, specialized tissue in the center of the heart helps form the tricuspid and mitral valves; it also plays a part in closing the lower part of the atrial septum and the top of the ventricular septum. When this tissue does not develop as it should, an *endocardial cushion defect* results. Sometimes the term *atrioventricular septal defect* is used to describe an endocardial cushion defect. *Atrioventricular canal defect* is also an appropriate term, because there is a wide opening, a freely flowing canal, between the left and right sides of the heart. The defect may be mild or moderate in its effects or extremely serious. In the severe form, a *complete atrioventricular canal defect*, heart failure may start in early infancy, and surgery is usually recommended before the first birthday to avoid complications from high pressure in the lungs. (Figure 6.1 shows a severe endocardial cushion defect, with the lower part of the atrial septum and the upper part of the ventricular septum missing. Treatment of complete atrioventricular canal defect is discussed in chapter 13.) Milder or partial forms of the defect, involving mainly the atrial septum, cause much less trouble, and surgery is usually performed during early childhood, before the child begins school.

Because the flow of blood through endocardial cushion defects is from the left side of the heart to the right, these defects are occasionally included with other septal defects, the *left-to-right shunts* discussed in chapter 4. There are good reasons to consider them as a separate group, however, as we do in this chapter. First, they develop differently: they

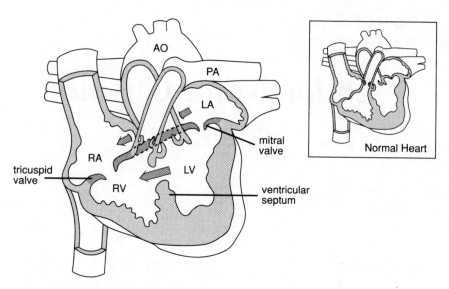

6.1. Endocardial Cushion Defect. In the severe form of the defect, a complete atrioventricular canal, there is a single large opening in the center of the heart; the *upper arrow* shows blood passing from the left atrium (*LA*) to the right (*RA*), the lower arrow from the left ventricle (*LV*) to the right (*RV*). Instead of two separate mitral and tricuspid valves, there is one large common valve, shown as a *dark shaded line* between the atria and the ventricles.

are caused not by abnormalities of flow during the development of the embryo's heart but by a specific, probably genetically controlled, failure of division of the specialized matrix tissue that forms the endocardial cushions. Second, they behave differently after birth because of the additional abnormalities of the mitral and tricuspid valves and the frequent association with Down syndrome.

Ostium Primum Atrial Septal Defect

In the mildest form of an atrioventricular canal defect the ventricular septum is almost normal; only the lower part of the atrial septum is missing, and there is usually also an abnormality of the mitral valve. The mitral valve appears to have a cleft in it; it fails to close completely with each heartbeat, allowing some blood to leak back from the left ventricle to the left atrium. Because the principal problem here is in the lower atrial septum, this is sometimes called an *ostium primum* type of atrial septal defect.

Between the most severe and the mildest forms of this anomaly are a number of *intermediate* atrioventricular canal defects; they vary in the size of the hole in the center of the heart and in the degree of severity of leaking or insufficiency of the mitral and tricuspid valves.

Complete Atrioventricular Canal Defect

In some children the development of the heart has been arrested at a very early stage. The specialized endocardial cushions in the center of the primitive heart have failed to grow and separate in a normal way. The heart has a major defect: there is a large open space in the center of the heart, and therefore blood can pass back and forth between the left and right atria and the left and right ventricles, as it is not intended to do. The lower atrial septum is missing and so is the upper part of the ventricular septum. As if this were not problem enough, the tricuspid valve, on the right, and the mitral valve, on the left, are incomplete and thus allow blood to leak back from the ventricles into the atria (figure 6.1).

Babies who have endocardial cushion defects may show a number of different symptoms:

- A heart murmur is usually, *but not always*, audible from birth.
- Feeding is slower than normal; the slowness increases between the ages of 1 and 6 months.
- Signs of heart failure—rapid breathing, slow growth, and sweating—may appear.
- Chest infections are frequent, sometimes leading to pneumonia.

Diagnosis can be surprisingly difficult because the heart murmur may not be loud. Occasionally the defect is found before birth by means of fetal echocardiography; after birth the defect is often found during evaluation of a newborn baby who has been recognized as having Down syndrome.

The heart murmur in such conditions is variable, but many other signs indicate that a serious heart problem exists. The baby's breathing is rapid, the heart is overactive, and the right ventricle can be felt to be enlarged and pumping too hard. An electrocardiogram shows an abnormal pattern seen in almost no other defect. An echo-Doppler shows the defect in the center of the heart and shows that the mitral and tricuspid valves are badly formed and leaky. Cardiac catheterization is sometimes recommended to permit the doctor to see the valves even more clearly and to measure the pressure in the lungs.

The delay in the onset of symptoms is related to changes in the small arteries of the lungs. Immediately after birth the pressure in the infant's lung arteries remains very high, so circulation, although abnormal, is balanced. Somewhere between one and six months after birth the pressure in the lung arteries falls somewhat, allowing blood to move from the left side of the heart into the right ventricle and the lungs. The heart rapidly enlarges, the lungs become more congested every day, and the baby becomes exhausted during feeding. The heart murmur usually becomes louder at the same time. In this precarious state, the baby is ultrasensitive to any viral illness that is going around. A particular virus known as the *respiratory syncytial virus* may invade the infant's congested lungs and lead to severe pneumonia, while the rest of the family experiences what seems like a cold or a mild attack of flu.

It is impossible to discuss complete atrioventricular canal defects without mentioning their very strong association with Down syndrome. More than 60 percent of all complete atrioventricular canal defects occur in infants with Down syndrome, and more than 30 percent of infants with Down syndrome have this defect. Because a heart murmur may be quite faint, any breathing difficulty the baby has can be mistakenly blamed on the characteristics of Down syndrome itself.

Atrioventricular Canal Defect with a Hypoplastic Ventricle

When one of the ventricles (usually the left) fails to grow properly before birth, the baby is born with both a small (hypoplastic) left ventricle and a complete atrioventricular canal defect. This atrioventricular canal defect with a hypoplastic ventricle is sometimes referred to as an "unbalanced atrioventricular canal," meaning there is no normal balance or ratio between the two ventricles. By any name, this is an extremely serious defect. Occasionally a Norwood type of operation will help, but successful treatment in such cases remains the exception.

Chapter 7

Other Congenital Heart Defects

Some of the congenital heart defects described in this chapter cause no trouble at all, but others are serious. All are very unusual. They are described here in some detail because the handbooks on congenital heart disease contain less information about them than about the more common defects. These unusual conditions include looping defects of the heart, such as dextrocardia; congenital abnormalities of the pulmonary veins and coronary arteries; and heart tumors. A few other very rare congenital defects do occur, but they are not included here.

Looping Defects

A looping defect of the heart occurs very early in development. In the normal looping process, the heart lies in the left side of the chest. Powerful genetic forces control this looping process and are responsible for the fact that nearly everyone's heart is located in the left side of the chest.

Some parts of the body are symmetrical and others are one-sided, or asymmetrical. There is a striking contrast between the asymmetry of the inside of the body (the left-sided heart, the right-sided liver) and the symmetry of the outside of the body (the limbs, the facial features, and the ears). Externally, our right and left sides are essentially mirror images. But inside, the heart is on the left, the liver on the right. There is only one appendix, and almost everyone knows that the appendix is in the right side of the lower abdomen. The asymmetry is programmed into the genetic function of development. Work with a special strain of mice in which the normal asymmetry has been disturbed has shown that there is a gene controlling place or position (*situs*). In the great majority of humans and mammals, the heart is in the left side of the chest, the liver in the right side of the abdomen. But in some, the position of the liver, stomach, and other abdominal organs is the opposite of normal (*situs inversus*, or turned around). Sometimes position is really mixed up, almost scrambled, with the liver in the center of the abdomen, the stomach misplaced, and even the appendix's place unpredictable. This condition is known as **heterotaxy**—that is, different or other than normal.

If the gene controlling the place of the abdominal organs is faulty or missing, chance takes over: half the hearts loop to the right, half to the left. In humans, looping defects are usually familial, although sometimes the family pattern is very difficult to track down. Many family studies suggest that the gene for abnormal position in humans is inherited (autosomal recessive). If parents have one child with abnormal position of one or more organs, there is approximately one chance in four that a later child will be similarly affected.

There are really only three basic types of looping problem, although a complicated language has grown up around them: *mirror-image dextrocardia, dextrocardia with abnormal heart,* and *heterotaxy.* Some writers include ventricular inversion (also called levo-transposition of the great arteries) under the heading of looping defects. We are not discussing this condition in detail, but include a story of a pioneer patient with such a heart problem in chapter 17.

Mirror-image dextrocardia

This is the simplest of the looping problems to understand. The name is really self-explanatory. In this situation (sometimes called *dextrocardia with situs inversus*) the heart is normal, except that it lies in the right side of the chest with the apex pointing to the right (figure 7.1). In true mirror-image dextrocardia, everything in the chest and abdomen is on the opposite side from usual: the appendix is on the left, the stomach on the right, the liver on the left, and so on: a mirror-image reversal of the normal arrangement.

Mirror-image dextrocardia first came to attention when routine chest X-rays began to be used in the 1920s and 1930s, when tuberculosis posed a significant public health hazard. X-ray surveys were done of

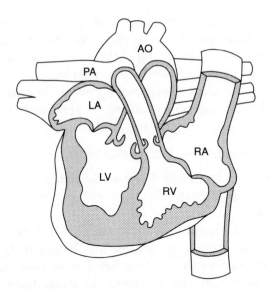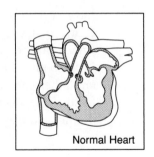

Normal Heart

7.1. Dextrocardia. In mirror image dextrocardia, shown here, the apex of the heart points to the right. The heart chambers, the left atrium (*LA*) and left ventricle (*LV*), the right atrium (*RA*) and right ventricle (*RV*) are all reversed, as in a mirror. The aorta (*AO*) and pulmonary artery (*PA*) connect with the appropriate ventricles. Usually the organs in the abdomen are also reversed (situs inversus), so that the liver lies on the left and the stomach on the right, the opposite of normal.

people reaching the age for army service and of people admitted to hospital for any reason. Radiologists soon realized that out there in the healthy population were some people whose organs were placed differently from those of other people. Two discoveries soon followed: first, a mirror-image arrangement was rare, appearing in only one in ten thousand routine X-rays; second, that this condition ran in families, in a recessive way—that is, both the father and mother had hearts on the left but carried the mirror-image gene, so that one in four of their children would have a right-sided heart and a left-sided appendix.

The idea of a mirror image attracted considerable interest outside the medical profession. Detective story writers thought up complicated plots involving almost identical twins, one a mirror image of the other, or a stab to the heart that failed because the heart was on the other side. In real life, people with this mirror-image arrangement sometimes derive amusement from watching to see whether examining doctors will notice which side the heart is on.

Although most children and adults with mirror-image dextrocardia have completely healthy, functioning hearts, it has been learned recently that some of them have abnormal cilia. Cilia are little moving fronds on the surface of the inside lining of the nostrils and elsewhere in the body. The normal motion of cilia keeps the secretions in the nose and other parts of the respiratory system moving; when the cilia are defective, the person has *Kartagener's syndrome*, or abnormal cilia syndrome, and may display severe respiratory symptoms.

Dextrocardia with abnormal heart

This condition is rare, but it is more common than mirror-image dextrocardia. About 2 infants in every 100 born with an abnormal heart also have dextrocardia.

The mere fact that the heart is on the "wrong" side does not prevent successful repair of any heart defect that may be found. The outlook depends on the inside structure of the heart itself. When the defect is a simple one, such as an atrial or ventricular septal defect, it can be repaired just as easily as if the heart were in the usual position. Most of the time, however, the defect is complex and involves an abnormal arrangement of the arteries leaving the heart. The arteries are transposed, but this is never a simple transposition; there is always a large ventricular septal defect, and often the ventricles cannot be distinguished from one another—there is really one big pumping chamber or "single ventricle." The child is usually cyanotic or blue from birth, and usually two or more staged operations are needed to restore circulation to as near normal as possible.

Heterotaxy

In the complicated situation of heterotaxy, the heart may be on the left or the right side and the abdominal organs are misplaced, often being in the midline rather than on one side or the other. In some heterotaxies the spleen is missing (*asplenia*) and in others there are many spleens (*polysplenia*), so sometimes the term *splenic syndrome* is used. "Sidedness" is also disturbed. Instead of two atria with different anatomy, the atria appear identical.

Right atrial isomerism (asplenia)

In babies born without a spleen, both atria resemble the right atrium. In addition, the septation of the heart and all the orderly sequence of conotruncal development are disturbed. Right atrial isomerism (asplenia) is one of the most serious of all congenital heart defects. The baby is intensely blue immediately after birth, owing to a complex of abnormalities. These vary in different babies, but usually include a large endocardial cushion defect (complete atrioventricular canal defect), transposition of the aorta and pulmonary artery, and severe pulmonary stenosis. As if all this were not enough, all the pulmonary veins often drain into the wrong side of the atrium. Remarkably, a few of these babies can be helped by a succession of operations, and some do very well. Because the spleen plays an important part in fighting infection, babies without a spleen need to be on continuous penicillin treatment to ward off meningitis caused by the pneumococcus and other bacteria.

The association between spleen abnormalities and heart defects was first described by Ivemark, so some medical texts describe heterotaxies under the heading of *Ivemark syndrome*. It is fair to say that heterotaxies are almost as difficult to read about as they are to describe and treat, partly because so many different words are used.

Left atrial isomerism (polysplenia)

When there are multiple spleens, both atria resemble the left atrium. Left atrial isomerism (polysplenia) is a much less serious problem than asplenia. Usually the heart defect is an atrial or ventricular septal defect with pulmonary stenosis. The pulmonary veins drain partly normally, partly abnormally. Most of these babies are only mildly blue and often all of the defects can be repaired in one operation, performed when the child is between 1 and 6 years of age.

Anomalies of the Pulmonary Venous Return

In the normal heart all four pulmonary veins enter the left atrium separately, two from the right lung and two from the left lung (figure 7.2). In abnormal or anomalous pulmonary venous return, some or all of the pulmonary veins connect to the right atrium instead of the left; sometimes they connect directly with the right atrium but more often they connect to a vein outside the heart, which then leads to the right atrium. How do the strange connections shown in figure 7.3 come about?

When the pulmonary veins are forming in the primitive lung bud of the embryo the atrium has not separated into two sides, and the small veins from the lung are very close to two large veins that drain into the right atrium. The veins grow toward the left atrium, an embryological process described as "targeted growth." If something happens

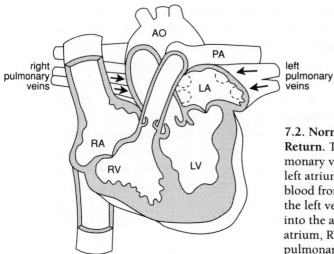

7.2. Normal Pulmonary Venous Return. The right and left pulmonary veins all connect with the left atrium (*LA*). Thus, oxygenated blood from the lungs passes into the left ventricle (*LV*) and then into the aorta (AO). (RA = right atrium, RV = right ventricle, PA = pulmonary artery)

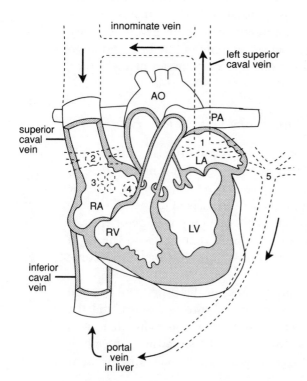

7.3. Abnormal Pulmonary Venous Return. All the pulmonary veins return to the right atrium (*RA*) by various routes. In (*1*), the most usual variant, the pulmonary veins join together behind the heart, drain upward, and eventually reach the right atrium via the superior caval vein. In (*2*), all the veins drain into the superior caval vein and in (*3*) and (*4*), directly into the right atrium. In (*5*), the pulmonary veins join behind the heart and drain downward to the liver, eventually reaching the right atrium via the inferior caval vein. (Partial pulmonary venous anomalies are not illustrated.)

to disturb this targeted growth—perhaps the embryo has a faulty gene, or a toxin causes a transient disturbance in embryo chemistry—the veins may miss the left side of the primitive atrium and end up joined to one of the body veins or connected directly to the right atrium.

We do not know exactly what makes the veins "target" the left atrium, but we think it likely that there is a form of chemical control, and that this control is under genetic influence. We do know that abnormalities in the connection of the pulmonary veins to the heart are more likely to happen if the lung is small or otherwise abnormal, and are particularly likely to occur when there is heterotaxy, a problem with right and left sidedness. A baby with no spleen or too many spleens will almost always have some abnormal connection of the pulmonary veins. These facts support the idea that some chemistry is involved in targeted growth: if the left side of the atrium is itself abnormal or misplaced, the usual targeting mechanisms fail, and the pulmonary veins connect to the nearest vein or atrium.

Total anomalous pulmonary venous return

Total anomalous pulmonary venous return is a serious defect, causing enlargement of the right heart chambers and usually requiring surgical repair early in infancy. In this condition, all the pulmonary veins connect wrongly, reaching the right atrium instead of the left. It often surprises people that the most frequent anomalous route (indicated by the number 1 in figure 7.3) looks the most complicated: the veins all join together behind the left atrium, and then course upward and across the chest before reaching the superior caval vein. This route is less bizarre during early life in the womb, because there is a large left-sided vein there (the left superior cardinal vein) ready to connect with the pulmonary veins if something disturbs their normal targeted growth into the left atrium.

Having all of the blood from the lungs, as well as the body, return to the right side of the heart causes rapid enlargement of the right-sided chambers of the heart. Some blood escapes from the right atrium to the left through a small atrial defect, but even so, the right side of the heart is under tremendous strain. Rapid breathing, difficulty in feeding, poor weight gain, and a heart murmur usually lead to early referral to a cardiologist.

Sometimes the veins from the lung are narrowed or obstructed as they enter the abnormal channel leading to the right atrium. When the veins drain down toward the liver (figure 7.3, number 5), they are often obstructed. In such babies rapid breathing and a blue color immediately after birth may lead doctors to suspect that spasm of the small lung arteries is causing high pressure in the lungs. It is easy to detect that the baby is seriously ill, but not always so easy to define that the veins of the lung are at fault. Even with Doppler-echocardiography, detecting the exact nature of the problem may be difficult at first.

Partial anomalies

Partial anomalies are not uncommon, and usually give rise to little difficulty. In a partial anomaly, only one or two of the pulmonary veins connect to the right atrium instead of the left. There are several different variations of this condition; in the most frequent variation, two veins from the right lung connect to the superior caval vein just as it joins the right atrium. In children who have this defect there is usually an opening between the right and left atrium, high up in the septum. This combination of abnormal venous return and atrial defect is called a *sinus venosus* type of atrial septal defect. As discussed in chapter 4, children with this defect have very few if any symptoms, and the problem is detected because a heart murmur leads to full cardiac evaluation. The defect can be repaired in early childhood, but unlike repair of most atrial septal defects, repair of a sinus venosus defect requires that a patch of pericardium or Gortex be applied to reroute the veins into the left atrium. The long-term outlook is good.

More rarely, the right lung is smaller than the left and the veins from the right lung join the inferior caval vein close to the diaphragm. The right-sided veins make a shadow on the chest X-ray that looks like a curved sword; this *scimitar syndrome* varies a great deal in severity, depending chiefly on the degree of underdevelopment of the right lung. When the lung is near normal size, the child's only problems are a heart murmur and an abnormal shadow on the chest X-ray. Repair of the defect, by rerouting the veins into the left atrium, can be done without difficulty in early childhood or even adulthood.

However, if the right lung is very small, there may be three additional problems. First, the lung may be subject to frequent infections, so that the infant is in and out of the hospital with pneumonia. Second, the heart is displaced into the right chest, and the left lung has to do most of the work of breathing. Third, and most serious, large abnormal arteries may lead from the aorta into the tiny right lung. This means the lung is not only too small but constantly flooded with too much blood under high pressure. Such babies may urgently need surgery in infancy to tie off the abnormal arteries; this surgery can be life-saving, but even after surgery the infant often grows slowly and is frailer than normal. We do not fully understand why this is so, but in its severe form the scimitar syndrome represents not a simple anomaly of the pulmonary veins but a complex heart-lung maldevelopment.

Coronary Artery Abnormalities

Normally, the right and left coronary arteries arise from the aorta and supply oxygen and nutrients to the heart (figure 7.4). There has been a great surge in the number of detailed X-ray pictures of the coronary artery tree since **coronary artery bypass surgery** became widely used. A surprising number of people who have been healthy into their fifties, or even their eighties, are found to have missing or misplaced coronary artery branches. This is not our topic, although it does point to a need for continuing work on coronary artery embryology and development. Here we will describe briefly some rare coronary defects that can lead to difficulty in infancy or childhood.

Anomalous origin of the left coronary artery from the pulmonary artery

An infant with anomalous origin of the left coronary artery from the pulmonary artery seems quite healthy at birth and usually has no heart murmur or anything to direct attention to the heart. During the early months of life, however, trouble begins. As the pressure in the lung arteries falls, blood begins to flow backward: it begins flowing from the aorta down the right coronary artery, in the normal way, but then flows back *up* the left coronary artery to the pulmonary artery (figure 7.5). This condition is often described as a "coronary steal," meaning that good oxygen-containing blood is being stolen from the heart muscle by the abnormal flow into the pulmonary artery.

The child's first symptom is usually difficulty in feeding. At somewhere between 3 and 6 months of age the infant stops feeding eagerly, and often cries and seems colicky after feeding only a few minutes. Sometimes during feeding the child sweats, struggles, and draws the knees up, suggesting that the infant is in severe pain. We believe that these babies feel the kind of agonizing pain felt by an older patient with **angina pectoris**. Other times the pain will be less obvious, but the baby's sweating, difficulty in feeding, and slow growth cause the parents to seek medical attention.

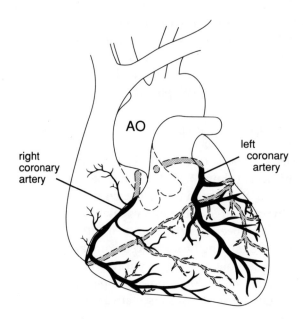

7.4. Coronary Arteries. Both coronary arteries normally arise from the aorta (*AO*) and divide into branches that spread out over the heart wall to supply the oxygen and nutrients needed for normal heart function.

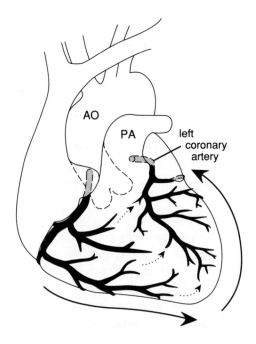

7.5. Anomalous Origin of the Left Coronary Artery from the Pulmonary Artery. Here the course of blood flow is from the aorta (*AO*) down the right coronary artery, then back up the left coronary artery to the pulmonary artery (*PA*). This course prevents the normal supply of oxygen and nutrients from reaching the left ventricle.

This condition can be a very difficult problem to recognize; many normal babies have episodes of being colicky, and only very, very occasionally is their discomfort caused by heart problems. The parents' account of the infant's sweating and pain may be the clues that alert the nurse or physician to the defect. Sometimes the enlargement of the heart can be detected when the physician examines the baby. Heart murmurs are very faint, so early detection by this means is not easy.

Once a heart problem is suspected, chest X-ray, EKG, and echo-Doppler studies will be helpful. The chest X-ray confirms that the heart, particularly the left ventricle, is larger than normal. The EKG may show a quite specific set of changes, exactly like those seen in a middle-aged person who is having a severe heart attack. This infarct pattern on the EKG occurs because the heart muscle of the left ventricle is getting insufficient oxygen and nutrients; the blood that should supply the muscle is going into the pulmonary artery is being "stolen." Even though the baby is only 2 or 3 months old, some of the muscle of the vital left ventricle is dead or dying. The echo-Doppler shows three important things: first, the enlargement of the right coronary artery, which has dilated in an effort to increase the flow of blood to the damaged heart; second, the extent of damage to the heart muscle (often seen); and third, the abnormal course of the blood flow back up into the pulmonary artery. Cardiac catheterization is sometimes needed if the echo-Doppler findings are not conclusive or if an additional defect is suspected.

Abnormal course of the left coronary artery

The left coronary artery usually comes off the left side of the aortic root (see figure 7.4). In perhaps one in a million people, it comes instead from the *right* side of the aorta and has to twist its way between the aorta and the pulmonary artery. Although this unusual course does not cause any heart murmur or anything that leads to a suspicion of heart disease, during strenuous exercise the artery may become twisted on itself, resulting in sudden severe chest pain. For some reason, possibly because teenagers exercise more strenuously, this happens most often in adolescence and seldom in early childhood. A combination of exercise electrocardiography and echo-Doppler testing can identify the problem. If a cardiac catheter test confirms the artery's abnormal course, surgery to reroute the coronary artery is usually recommended, because the defect occasionally leads to the sudden death of an otherwise healthy teenager engaged in strenuous exercise. Surgical treatment may relieve the problem completely, provided that the heart muscle has not already been too badly damaged.

Fistulas

A fistula is an abnormal channel, or communication, between two structures that are not ordinarily joined.

Coronary artery fistula

A *coronary artery fistula* is an abnormal communication between one of the coronary arteries and the inside of a ventricle or atrium. Usually a loud and unusual heart murmur is heard; thus the condition generally is noticed by the pediatrician and so comes quickly to the attention of a cardiologist. If the fistula is quite large, the heart may become enlarged or signs of heart failure may appear.

In most babies this defect can be recognized on an echo-Doppler test, but generally a cardiac catheter test is performed so the surgeon can be certain of the best approach to take. If the fistula is very small surgical repair is not considered necessary, but the usual treatment is surgical and is very successful. In surgery the fistula is closed where it enters the heart chamber, usually with a small patch, so little if any damage is done to the coronary artery itself. Children who have this operation can become as active as normal children.

Arteriovenous fistula of the vein of Galen

An abnormal communication between an artery and a vein, known as an *arteriovenous fistula*, can be present before birth and may be discovered by a fetal echocardiogram; it can also occur almost anywhere in the body, but is found most often in the brain and sometimes in the liver. If the fistula is large, the baby can develop heart failure even before birth.

The most usual fistula, a cerebral arteriovenous fistula of the vein of Galen, lies between the arteries and veins inside the brain. A baby born with this problem has a large heart and becomes ill with heart failure very rapidly, as blood rushes through the abnormal communication in the center of the brain. It is an extremely serious problem. Once the defect is recognized, from the heart murmur and from echo-Doppler tests, treatment is attempted by specialists in neurology; some infants have been helped by the insertion of tiny coils into the artery that feeds the fistula, in an effort to close off the abnormal channel. Successful treatment is, so far, infrequent. Fistulas elsewhere in the body can more often be treated effectively, either by surgery or by insertion of balloons or coils in the catheterization laboratory.

Tumors of the Heart (Rhabdomyomas)

Most heart tumors in infants are caused by clusters of overgrown muscle cells, known as *rhabdomyomas*. These benign tumors are nearly always a sign that the baby has a neurological disorder called *tuberous sclerosis*. Because fetal echocardiography is now widely used, many of these tumors are discovered before birth. A few lead to obstruction of one of the heart valves and need surgery after birth, but most require no treatment and become smaller as the baby grows. The baby with tuberous sclerosis needs careful follow-up.

Oncocytic Cardiomyopathy

Oncocytic cardiomyopathy, a disorder called by many different names, is somewhere in a gray zone between heart muscle disease and an unusual heart tumor. In this condition there are tiny collections of cells in the wall of the ventricle that can set off abnormal heart rhythms. A baby with this problem may have repeated attacks of rapid heart rate (**tachycardia**) and may respond poorly to the usual medications. Specialized catheter tests can pinpoint the exact location of the abnormal cells in the ventricle: treatment, which in some cases has been remarkably successful, consists of surgical removal or freezing. In most cases, the child will then grow normally.

Ectopia Cordis

In ectopia cordis the heart grows partly or even completely on the outside of the chest wall. It is usually also badly formed in some other way, usually with a defect resembling tetralogy of Fallot. This is perhaps the only heart defect that can be diagnosed with no special skill or knowledge: there is no mistaking it. It is rarely successfully treated by surgery; fortunately, the defect is rare.

Most rare congenital heart problems can be treated surgically when necessary. As new knowledge is gained about normal heart development, many rare defects are beginning to be understood, and even greater successes in treatment should follow in the next decade. The gene for heterotaxy has been discovered in the mouse model, and this discovery has given researchers a great incentive to look closely at the genes that control the looping of the human heart. Some babies with total anomalous pulmonary venous return have an abnormality of chromosome 22; this discovery is stimulating research into the genes that control the targeted growth of the normal pulmonary veins toward the left atrium. As for the coronary arteries, much still needs to be learned about their normal development and why some arteries are more prone than others to atherosclerosis in middle age. Rare defects can sometimes provide significant clues to common and severe problems.

Chapter 8

Acquired Heart Problems

Most heart problems in children are a consequence of congenital heart defects—heart defects that occur before birth. A variety of problems, generally less complex than congenital defects—some mild and requiring no treatment, some moderate, and some severe—are the result not of a defect that occurs before birth but of a problem that develops after birth. The structure of the heart is normal and no congenital defect is present, but some problem arises later to cause concern about the child's heart. Most often, this later problem is the appearance of a heart murmur, an additional sound or noise between the two normal heart sounds, lub and dup. Sometimes this murmur is the result of a congenital abnormality, such as an atrial septal defect, but most often a newly detected murmur in a child over two years old is "innocent," meaning that it requires no treatment and no restriction of normal play or activity. (Innocent murmurs and murmurs caused by mitral valve prolapse are discussed in chapter 9.)

Heart problems that occur after birth—those discussed in this chapter—include arrhythmias, cardiomyopathy, rheumatic heart disease, and Kawasaki syndrome. Arrhythmias (abnormal rhythms of the heart) can appear even before birth, but most do not pose a problem until infancy or childhood. Cardiomyopathy, or disease of the heart muscle, can be caused by a genetic disorder or it can develop following a viral or other infection. Rheumatic heart disease can be a complication of rheumatic fever, an acute inflammation of the joints and heart following a **streptococcal infection** of the throat. Kawasaki syndrome, also known as **mucocutaneous lymph node syndrome**, occurs as an illness of young children that occasionally leads to damage to the heart muscle or the coronary arteries. These heart problems vary greatly in severity, but all can be treated.

Arrhythmias

In a healthy child the heart rate varies with age and with level of activity, but the rhythm is regular. To be more accurate, the rhythm is not absolutely regular, like a metronome or ticking clock, but varies slightly with breathing. You can test this by taking a deep breath—notice that the heartbeat is a little faster when you are inhaling than when you are exhaling. This variation with breathing (sinus arrhythmia), which is more obvious in young children than in adults, is a sign of a healthy heart. The electrocardiogram of a person who has a normal rhythm of the heart is said to show *normal sinus rhythm*; the heart's natural **pacemaker** which controls the rhythm of the heart, is in the **sinus**, or **sinoatrial node**. The node is a small focus of specialized heart muscle cells lying just where the superior vena cava joins the right atrium. It is richly supplied with nerve endings and is exquisitely sensitive to the body's needs and to messages from the nervous system (see figure 8.1). An impulse arising in the sinus node passes through the atrium to the **atrioventricular node** at the upper part of the ventricular septum. From there, the electrical impulse passes down a bundle of specialized muscle fibers on either side of the ventricular septum and then fans out over the ventricular walls. Thus, the impulse follows an orderly sequence. When the orderly sequence is disturbed, the regular rhythm of the heart is lost and arrhythmia occurs.

Arrhythmias of children include

- *Tachycardias,* which produce a persistent rapid heart rate and abnormal rhythm.
- *Bradycardias,* which produce a persistent slow heart rate and abnormal rhythm.
- *Others,* including *long QT syndrome,* a rare and dangerous condition, and **extrasystoles** (premature contractions), a common and usually harmless condition.

Abnormal heart rhythms vary a great deal in their impact on the child and the family. Most do not require treatment, but a few require prolonged medication and sometimes even surgical management.

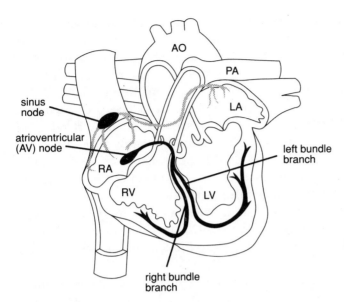

**8.1.
Heart Rhythm:
Normal Conducting
System.** The normal
electrical impulse of
the heart arises in the
sinus node and spreads
through the right (*RA*)
and left atrium (*LA*) to
the atrioventricular node.
From there it passes
down the specialized
bundles running in the
septum between the
right (*RV*) and left
ventricle (*LV*) and
spreads out over the
ventricles.

Tachycardias

It is quite normal for the heart rate of a child to rise (to 200, or even
more) after vigorous exercise. But if the rate *remains* high (at over 180
beats per minute in infants or 130 beats in children), even during rest
or sleep, it nearly always means that the impulse is not arising normally in the sinus node but either is arising in some other area of the
heart or is somehow being conducted abnormally. The two most frequent types of tachycardia (persistent too-rapid heartbeat) in children
are ectopic atrial tachycardia and reentry tachycardia.

Ectopic atrial tachycardia. *Ectopic* means "out of place." In this form of
tachycardia, an abnormal focus of scar tissue in the atrium takes over
the role of pacemaker from the sinus node. This new pacemaker lacks
the proper network of nerve endings that make the sinus node sensitive to the body's needs, and the ectopic focus continues to fire off at a
fixed rate, like a runaway car without brakes.

Reentry tachycardia. In some children there is an extra bundle of conducting tissue between the atrium and the ventricle of the heart. The
heart impulse starts off normally, in the sinus node, but then travels
down to the ventricle by way of this accessory bundle, bypassing the
atrioventricular node, which usually acts as a secondary regulator of

the heart rate. From the ventricle, the impulse now passes back up to the atrium by way of the normal bundle branch and then back down again to the ventricle. This process sets up a rapid rhythm called a *reentry tachycardia*, because the impulse reenters the atrium and does not follow the normal orderly sequence. The term *Wolff-Parkinson-White syndrome* is used when the accessory bundle produces a characteristic pattern on the child's EKG between episodes of rapid heart rate. The child with this syndrome is completely normal most of the time, and the diagnosis is made from the characteristic change on the EKG, performed as part of a routine checkup or after an episode of tachycardia. The syndrome is named after three physicians, Drs. Harold Wolff and Paul Dudley White of the United States and Sir John Parkinson of Great Britain, who recognized in the 1920s that individuals with a certain unusual electrocardiographic pattern often have attacks of tachycardia.

In both of these types of tachycardia the normal sensitive controls of the sinus node no longer work, and the heartbeat is persistently fast. Although the heart muscle has great energy reserves, it will not tolerate extreme tachycardia indefinitely, and heart failure may develop.

Two other forms of atrial tachycardia, known as *atrial fibrillation* and *atrial flutter*, are much rarer in children than adults; in both arrhythmias the atrium beats fast and irregularly. Treatment is needed urgently, often involving more than one medication. Usually a child with such an abnormal rhythm has some severe congenital heart defect, unlike the children with more common types of tachycardia.

Ventricular tachycardia. Ventricular tachycardias, caused by an abnormal focus in the ventricle, are more dangerous than atrial tachycardias. Ventricular tachycardia may be detected when an irregular pulse is noted during a pediatric examination. An EKG will show a succession of more than three heartbeats arising from the ventricle without a normal P wave before each beat (see figure 2.7). When episodes of tachycardia are found in this way, and the child has no symptoms, a decision about treatment can be quite difficult, because sometimes the side effects of treatment are more troublesome than the changes on the EKG.

In other children, ventricular tachycardia may lead to severe palpitations, dizziness, or even passing out during or after exertion. The normal heart rhythm is restored by using electroconversion (passing an electric current through the body). A number of tests may be needed before the best combination of medications to prevent any further such attacks is found. In most children with ventricular tachycardia no other abnormality of the heart is detected even after multiple tests, sometimes including cardiac catheterization. In a few teenagers the tachycardia may arise from an abnormally thin area in the right ventricular wall, called *arrhythmogenic right ventricle*. In other children, ventricular tachycardia may be a complication of a congenital heart defect, occurring either before or after open-heart surgery. At one time it was seen in a number of children after repair of tetralogy of Fallot, but it seems to be decreasing in this group now that heart surgery is performed at a much younger age than in the past (see chapter 12).

Attacks of ventricular tachycardia that do result in symptoms such as fainting (syncope) are dangerous, because they may progress to the point where the child has a weak and ineffective heartbeat known as *ventricular fibrillation*. Any child who has an episode of ventricular tachycardia needs careful evaluation in a heart center that specializes in childhood arrhythmias. In addition to prescribing and monitoring any necessary medications, the health team at the center will help the family reach a decision about the child's participation in sports and strenuous activities. The team will also be able to determine whether there is an abnormal focus in the ventricle that can be treated by special catheter techniques or by surgery (usually surgery is advised only if medications have been unsuccessful). Children with this disorder, like children with congenital heart defects, must be considered as unique individuals. The health team, the child, and the family need to have a well-constructed triangle of understanding.

Bradycardias

Bradycardias are abnormally slow heart rhythms. Although healthy teenage athletes may have heart rates as slow as 40 beats per minute, in newborn babies a rate persistently below 100 is unusual, and a rate below 60 may mean the normal conduction through the heart is faulty. *Congenital complete heart block* may be present, with the atrium and the ventricle beating separately, each "marching to a different drummer." Congenital heart block in a baby with an otherwise normal heart has been found to be caused by abnormal Ro antibodies that have crossed the placenta during pregnancy and damaged the infant's developing conduction system. Pacemaker treatment may be needed. Sometimes the baby also has a complex heart defect; more often there is no other problem in the heart.

Abnormally slow heart rhythms in older children that are not related to an advanced degree of physical training are usually caused by poor functioning of the sinus node (*sinus node dysfunction*). In this condition, sometimes called "sick sinus syndrome," runs of rapid heart rate may alternate with very slow rates.

Occasionally an episode of fainting is the first indication of trouble; more often an irregular heart rhythm is detected during a physical examination. Depending on how slow the rate becomes during sleep, implantation of a pacemaker may be required (see chapter 14).

Arrhythmias may also occur as side effects of drugs, both prescription medications and street drugs such as cocaine. They may also be a complication in teenagers who use liquid protein diets for weight reduction.

Other Arrhythmias

Long QT syndrome. Long QT syndrome is an unusual condition in which the child shows no sign of illness, except in rare instances when the syndrome is associated with congenital deafness. A sudden fainting episode during exercise or when the child is acutely stressed or excited may be the first clue. The syndrome is very likely to run in a family.

This syndrome is one of electrical instability of the heart. If a new electrical impulse reaches the ventricle during the T wave—the so-called vulnerable period—it may set off a run of ventricular beats leading to ventricular tachycardia. This is especially likely to happen during stress. Some evidence suggests that there is an imbalance of the sympathetic nerve supply to the heart.

Whatever the exact mechanism by which the long QT syndrome leads to ventricular tachycardia, most children with the syndrome require treatment. Treatment is particularly urgent if there is a family history of long QT syndrome with fainting spells or sudden death, or if the child has experienced faintness or has passed out during or after exercise or stress. The condition is usually treated with a medication known as a beta-blocker, which slows down the response of the heart rate to stress or exertion and makes extra heartbeats less likely to fall into the vulnerable period. It is essential that such medication (or even surgery) be prescribed and monitored from a heart center that specializes in childhood arrhythmias. (For an example of a family and child with this rare but significant heart problem, see chapter 11.)

Extrasystoles. An extrasystole, or premature beat, is an impulse that arises before the next regular beat is due. It is extra, meaning that it occurs in addition to the normal regular beats that arise from the sinus node. It is premature in the sense that it comes on earlier than the next expected beat. It arises from an ectopic focus, that is, from a place in the heart other than the sinus node. Almost everyone has experienced such an extra beat, perhaps after drinking a lot of coffee or during times of stress. Sometimes the beat feels like a "thud" in the chest: after several such beats in a row a teenager may say, "It felt like my heart was jumping out of my chest." Sometimes the extra beat is followed by a pause: "It felt like my heart stopped, like it skipped a beat." Extrasystoles may be detected when a child goes for a regular checkup, but teenagers may find them uncomfortable and worrisome enough to bring them to the attention of parents or doctors.

The extra beats arise in the heart muscle—sometimes in the atrium, often in the ventricle. Usually only ventricular extrasystoles are considered for treatment. The focus they come from is probably an area of scarring, where there's been some local damage to a heart muscle cell.

Cardiomyopathy: Disease of the Myocardium

Cardiomyopathy (figure 8.2) is increasingly recognized as an important, although rare, problem in childhood. The muscle of the heart (the myocardium) is a wonderfully complex structure, consisting of bands of fibers of myofibrils that contract to form the normal strong, regular heartbeat. In some children, about three in ten thousand, the myocardium may become damaged and cardiomyopathy develops.

There are many possible causes of cardiomyopathy. Most instances are thought to follow viral infection. Although most viral infections of the heart are followed by complete recovery, in some children a prolonged disease of the heart muscle may follow. The extent of the damage depends in part on the severity of the original viral illness and in part on how the body itself responds to attack (the "immune response"). Some forms of dilated and hypertrophic cardiomyopathy may be a result of gene abnormalities. With intensive research now under way into the genetic basis for the different types of cardiomyopathy, development of means of prevention seems likely in the years to come. A child who has a prolonged period of rapid heart rate from an ectopic

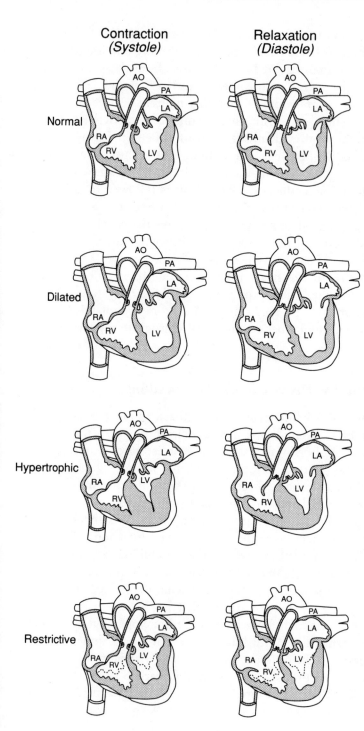

Contraction
(Systole)

Relaxation
(Diastole)

Normal

Dilated

Hypertrophic

Restrictive

8.2.
Cardiomyopathy.
In the *normal* heart the right (*RV*) and left ventricle (*LV*) are smaller in systole (when the heart is contracting) than in diastole, when the heart relaxes. The heart chambers are of normal size and the muscle squeeze, or contraction, is strong. In *dilated* cardiomyopathy the ventricles, particularly the left ventricle, are dilated and the contraction is weak so that the size of the ventricle shows little change between systole and diastole. The heart does not empty properly. In *hypertrophic* cardiomyopathy the ventricular muscle is thick, particularly the ventricular septum, and although the heart can squeeze well, it cannot relax normally; this inability to relax leads to even greater hypertrophy. In *restrictive* cardiomyopathy the inner lining or endocardium of both ventricles is thickened (shown by a *dotted line* inside LV and RV), also leading to failure of relaxation of the heart in diastole.

atrial rhythm may also develop cardiomyopathy, which will resolve once the rhythm returns to normal. Sometimes no cause can be found.

The treatment of these heart muscle problems is diverse. The diseased myocardium often responds to some of the newer heart medications. When the heart muscle is hopelessly damaged, heart transplant is now an accepted alternative (see chapter 13).

Viral myocarditis

Viral myocarditis is an inflammation of the heart muscle caused by a viral infection. The inflammation may heal completely, leaving no sign of damage, or it may result in mild scarring.

Almost any virus can affect the myocardium. The Coxsackie virus is among those most frequently found in severe viral myocarditis. HIV, which causes AIDS, can also lead to severe cardiomyopathy.

Dilated cardiomyopathy

In dilated cardiomyopathy the heart muscle is weak and beats or contracts poorly, and the cavity of the heart is enlarged or dilated (figure 8.2). This kind of cardiomyopathy may follow viral myocarditis, or it may be caused by toxins or drugs or by other factors not yet understood. Alcohol is the most usual cause of dilated cardiomyopathy in adults; in children viral infection is a common cause. Drugs used to treat leukemia or other childhood cancers can be the culprit.

Cardiomyopathy may also be a complication of diseases of the nervous system such as Friedreich's ataxia or childhood muscle disorders such as Duchenne's muscular dystrophy.

Hypertrophic cardiomyopathy

In hypertrophic cardiomyopathy the wall of the ventricle is thickened (hypertrophied). In the most usual form, illustrated in figure 8.2, the septum, or wall between the ventricles, is much thicker than the rest of the left ventricle; it is sometimes called asymmetric septal hypertrophy for this reason. More rarely, both walls of the left ventricle are equally thickened; this is described as concentric ventricular hypertrophy.

In contrast to dilated cardiomyopathy, in hypertrophic cardiomyopathy the thick muscle can beat or contract normally, but it does not relax properly; increasing overwork and increasing hypertrophy are the result. The ventricle does not fill properly. It is rather like a person who, by continuous weightlifting, has developed enormous biceps, and become muscle-bound. Eventually, late in the course of the disease, the ventricle may dilate. In other cases, the overworked muscle contracts irregularly, the blood supply from the coronary arteries is not enough to supply the thickened muscle, and chest pain and arrhythmias result, with a risk of sudden death.

The condition of asymmetric septal hypertrophy, the most usual form of hypertrophic cardiomyopathy, usually runs in a family. Its cause is under active study. It is possible that it begins as an abnormality of the sympathetic nervous supply to the heart, causing progressive irregular muscle cell growth even before birth. Recent research suggests that the calcium channels inside the muscle cells of the heart may be the site of the problem, presumably because of a fault in one of the genes controlling the transmission of calcium into and out of the heart cell. Localization of the responsible gene or genes is already in sight.

Other cardiomyopathies

In other cases the chemistry or metabolism of the myocardium is faulty. *Pompe's disease* (glycogen storage disease of the heart), *congenital lactic acidosis*, and one type of *carnitine deficiency* are all in this group. These *metabolic* types of cardiomyopathy usually involve a deficiency of an enzyme that is necessary for normal chemical reactions in the heart. Both parents may carry an abnormal gene but have no heart difficulty; their child, however, inherits two abnormal genes, one from each parent, and may have severe progressive cardiomyopathy. For some of these children, including those with carnitine deficiency, the missing enzyme can be supplied through medication.

The heart muscle can also be affected by nutritional deficiency. Although this problem is almost unknown in the Western world, in areas of famine, lack of vitamin B may lead to beriberi heart disease, a disease that responds to proper diet and vitamin B. In certain parts of Africa poor nutrition plays a role in a severe cardiomyopathy involving thickening of the endocardium (the inner lining of the heart) and a smaller than normal heart cavity. The heart is unable to fill properly, and fluid accumulates throughout the body. In this *restrictive* cardiomyopathy (figure 8.2) the heart's response to improved diet is slow and disappointing.

Heart muscle problems can thus be a consequence of other severe diseases, a number of them preventable. Heart disease caused by malnutrition can be prevented by an adequate diet, but an adequate diet is not available in the parts of the world plagued by famine, and malnutrition rates are rising. The cardiomyopathy of AIDS, which is affecting infants born to HIV-positive mothers, is preventable in theory but difficult to prevent in practice. As we turn our attention to issues of child health—nationally and internationally, through UNICEF and other health agencies—problems like these should pass, like bubonic plague, into the pages of medical history. But this eventuality will take time and intense dedication and research.

Rheumatic Heart Disease

Acute rheumatic fever, once a common and devastating disease of childhood and still a major scourge in many Third World countries, has sharply declined in the West. Rheumatic fever generally affects children between 2 and 16 years of age after a throat infection by a Group A streptococcus virus. For the disease to occur, the child must have a throat infection with a particular subtype or strain of streptococcus, and the child must be susceptible to rheumatic fever. The child with rheumatic fever develops joint pain and swelling and an inflammation of the heart; the inflammation is most severe in the mitral and aortic valves and around the heart. Although the streptococcus does not infect the heart directly, it causes the body's immune system to produce antibodies, and these in turn inflame the heart tissue. There is still no effective vaccine for streptococcus.

Why is one child susceptible to this illness and another not? Despite volumes of research the answer is not in. Overcrowding, poverty, and youth contribute. There is some familial tendency, and there are some clues that immune system genes are involved—that the body's defenses against infection are not intact.

A few years ago rheumatic fever seemed to have disappeared in the United States and in Western Europe. The dramatic decline began even before the discovery of penicillin in the 1940s. With improved and less crowded housing, and with early treatment of streptococcal throat infections (which can occur repeatedly), the disease seemed almost gone. In the 1980s a few small clusters of rheumatic fever appeared again in several cities in the United States, but they were far less severe than cases seen in the past.

In the past, children with rheumatic fever were kept in bed for many weeks on aspirin or steroid treatment while the inflammation slowly healed. Now, bed rest is prescribed for only a week or two, and recovery is much more rapid. About two-thirds of the time the heart heals completely, but sometimes the inflammation that follows the throat infection causes the mitral valve to become insufficient, allowing blood to leak back into the left atrium with each heartbeat. Or the scarring of the mitral valve may lead to stenosis, or narrowing of the valve. Mitral stenosis or other valvar problems may require surgery. Recently stenotic valves in some children have been opened up by balloon catheterization, a great advance in treatment but not useful if the valve itself is insufficient.

One attack of rheumatic fever makes a child susceptible to another attack if a new streptococcal throat infection occurs. Therefore, to prevent further streptococcal infection, children who have had one attack of rheumatic fever are advised to take penicillin until they are at least 18 years of age.

Kawasaki Syndrome

Kawasaki syndrome begins as an acute illness in a young child, usually between 1 and 4 years old. The cause is as yet unknown. A high fever, extreme irritability, a red tongue and lips, conjunctivitis, swollen lymph glands in the neck, and a rash are followed a few days later by peeling of the fingers and toes. Some children develop an acute inflammation of the heart that resembles viral myocarditis. *Aneurysms of the coronary arteries* may form. Most of them shrink and disappear, but a few remain; if they rupture, sudden death may occur weeks or months after other signs of illness have long gone. However, early treatment with injections of immune globulin, followed by a course of aspirin, prevents aneurysms in nearly all affected children. Some children sustain damage to the lining of the coronary arteries that will later predispose them to coronary artery atherosclerosis. (The American Heart Association has an excellent booklet on this unusual and troublesome disorder.)

As congenital heart defects are more and more often successfully repaired in infancy, increasing attention is turning to heart problems that develop later, such as arrhythmias and cardiomyopathies. The myocardium is a complicated structure, and it has only recently become possible to study the chemical pathways that are used each time a fiber of heart muscle contracts. Because heart muscle cells can now be grown outside the body, researchers are beginning to identify some of the genes that contribute to growth of the heart and that control some of the chemical pathways needed for normal heart rhythm. This kind of research, known as *molecular biology*, is already providing clues to which genes are involved in one form of hypertrophic cardiomyopathy. In the next few decades, understanding and prevention of many myocardial disorders and rhythm abnormalities should lead to better health and growth for children everywhere.

Part III

THE
TREATMENT OF
HEART DEFECTS

Chapter 9

Problems That Require No Treatment

Approximately 1 of every 100 babies born has a heart defect. Fortunately, about one-third of the defects are so mild that they require no treatment at all. Sometimes a heart problem present at birth disappears as the child grows. For example, many small defects in the ventricular septum close by themselves over the first year or two of life. It is estimated that over one-third of small ventricular septal defects close and the murmur they caused in infancy disappears. Some atrial septal defects also close, perhaps one in ten of all those present at birth. Small septal defects are much more likely to close than large ones, and almost all closures happen before 2 years of age. Other conditions that usually require no treatment include innocent heart murmurs and mild congenital right- and left-heart flow defects.

A few of the heart problems that appear after birth, such as mitral valve prolapse (MVP) and extra heartbeats (extrasystoles), also need no treatment.

Several cases of such harmless conditions are reviewed in this chapter. No conotruncal defects or endocardial cushion defects are included here, because all conotruncal defects and almost all endocardial cushion defects are serious and require surgery. Treatment of these defects is discussed in chapters 10 and 12.

Innocent Heart Murmurs

Tommy J. was a particularly treasured little boy. His parents had waited until they were in their thirties to have a family. His

135

mother had had an amniocentesis and two echo tests during pregnancy because of early bleeding and, later, a suspicion of slow fetal growth. At birth Tommy was normal, and he grew into a fine, active 5-year-old. He was doing well in kindergarten. Shortly after his fifth birthday he went for an extra checkup following a rather severe head cold. The pediatrician listened to his heart for longer than usual. Mrs. J., who was very observant, asked if anything was wrong. "No, he seems fine. It's just that I hear a murmur, an extra sound over his heart. We often hear innocent murmurs at his age. Nothing to worry about. If I still hear it in another month or two, we'll talk about whether he needs to see a pediatric cardiologist or have any tests." He gave Mrs. J. a booklet on innocent heart murmurs to take home.

The booklet was clear and reassuring, but Tommy's parents were anxious. One of their neighbors, a 42-year-old with a family history of cholesterol problems, had died recently while out jogging. The J. family understood that there was no link between their neighbor's tragedy and the newly discovered murmur in Tommy's heart, but somehow even a suspicion of heart disease made them hover over Tommy and worry when he played actively.

Tommy's parents did not want to wait a month or more before making sure his heart was normal, and they made an appointment with a pediatric cardiologist, who checked Tommy two weeks later. She confirmed that the heart murmur sounded innocent; in addition, the electrocardiogram and echo-Doppler study were both completely normal. As Tommy and his parents looked at the echo on the videotape, the cardiologist showed them the normal heart valves opening and closing. She explained that the test confirmed that he had no "holes," or septal defects in his heart. She said, "He's as healthy as he looks. His heart is as wonderful as he is!"

Tommy's parents were told that he could be expected to lead a normal life and that he could take part in sports without any restrictions. He did not need any further checkups by a cardiologist.

Many parents have never read about innocent heart murmurs in any of the books and magazine articles published for parents. In the past, when some heart defects went undetected even into adult life, a great deal of attention was devoted to warning parents and physicians to be on the alert for defects; little was written about normal variations.

A principal purpose of this book is to help parents understand the developing heart and its variations during childhood, not only defects that require care but also findings such as innocent heart murmurs that need cause no concern.

Heart murmurs are common in children. Most of these innocent (that is, normal) heart murmurs are caused by blood vibrating as it flows through the heart. These vibrations are similar to the sounds made when the water tap is turned on and reverberations echo throughout the house. A pediatrician or family physician will usually recognize that these murmurs are of no concern and will reassure a worried parent. If the physician is not certain of this, he or she may refer the child to a pediatric cardiologist for evaluation and confirmation. When heart murmurs are normal, they pose no problem for the child. Follow-up visits will not be needed and the child's life expectancy and activities will be normal.

Some children who are born with normal hearts later show symptoms or findings that suggest the possibility that a heart problem has developed. Usually, the pediatrician will hear a new sound or murmur, a sound either that was not heard in infancy or that sounded faint in infancy and was expected to disappear. Occasionally such a murmur is caused by a congenital heart defect, but much more often it is one of the innocent murmurs of childhood.

Tommy's story prompts several questions. The question most often asked—"What exactly *is* a heart murmur?"—is difficult to answer briefly. In everyday life we think of a murmur as a soft and pleasant hum of voices.

Innocent heart murmurs, sometimes called *functional* or *normal murmurs*, are not a sign of heart disease. Indeed, some such murmur can be heard over the heart or the neck veins in almost half of all normal children at some time during childhood. They are usually first heard when a child is between 2 and 6 years old. Most of them become softer as the child grows and disappear by adulthood. But when parents hear the words *heart murmur*, they are often uneasy; they may be bothered by a number of questions after they get home, particularly if the visit to the doctor has been a hurried one and if they have not fully understood what was going on. Among their questions are these:

- What is a heart murmur?
- Why did no one hear my child's murmur before now?

- How can you be sure my child's heart is really okay?
- Will my child be able to live a normal life? Can he or she be active in sports, for example?

A heart murmur is caused by turbulent blood flow. It is an extra sound or noise heard between the normal first and second heart sounds. Even if you have never listened through a stethoscope, you probably have heard the lub-dup, lub-dup, lub-dup of heart sounds on taped recordings used on medical TV programs. Lub, the first sound, is caused by the contraction of the heart muscle and closure of the mitral valve; dup-p, the second sound, is caused by the closure of the aortic and pulmonary valves (see figure 2.7). The actual flow of blood through the heart produces a soft "whooshing" sound, normally too faint to hear through a stethoscope on the chest wall. If blood flow is more turbulent than usual, however, it causes a murmur or whoosh between lub and dup, a vibrating sort of noise, rather like water flowing through the pipes in a house. A murmur would always be recorded in every normal heart, child or adult, if a sensitive stethoscope were passed on a catheter into the pulmonary artery. The innocent murmur of childhood is the normal murmur amplified.

The most common innocent murmur, *Still's murmur* (named after the pediatrician who first described it), is caused by turbulent flow in the left ventricle of a young child's active heart. One interesting recent study has suggested that this turbulence arises when the aortic root is a little smaller than average, resulting in a swirling or turbulence of flow as blood passes from the left ventricle into the aorta. The murmur has a twanging or vibratory quality but is not very loud, and it varies as the child moves and breathes. The physician hears it most clearly over the lower part of the left chest, close to the sternum or breastbone. The murmur may be louder than usual when the output of the flow from the heart is increased, as it is when the child has a fever or anemia.

Other, less common but also innocent, murmurs may sometimes be heard over the upper chest and pulmonary artery (*benign pulmonary outflow murmur*); over the carotid artery (*carotid bruit*), or over the veins of the neck (*venous hum*) (see figure 9.1). Parents may well be perplexed that these innocent heart murmurs are identified in early childhood rather than in infancy. Tommy's parents had been relieved that the difficult days of teething and colic were past when suddenly the pediatrician heard this new sound! In Tommy's case, the murmur had become easier to hear at age 5 than when he was younger, probably

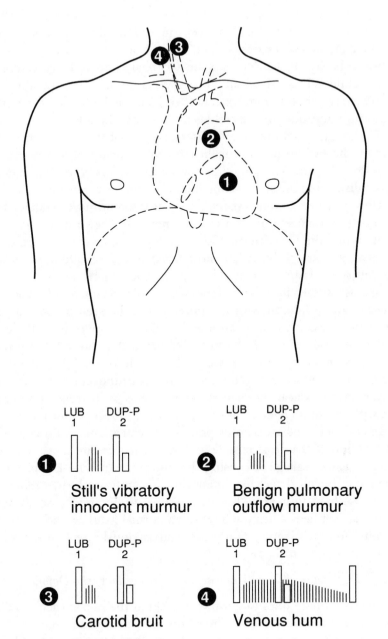

9.1. Innocent Murmurs of the Heart.

for one of two reasons: first, the heart rate of an older child is slower, and the child is less restless; second, some heart defects are hard to diagnose in babies. Pediatricians make a special effort to listen carefully when a child is between about 2 and 5 years for any hint of a mild defect. Thus, easier and more concentrated listening both may play a part in finding a murmur when a child is no longer an infant.

The gradual diminution and disappearance of most innocent murmurs by the early teens is probably the consequence of less turbulent blood flow. At the same time, the child's chest wall is becoming thicker, further distancing the stethoscope from any soft heart murmurs.

How sure can Tommy's parents be that the murmur the doctor has heard is truly innocent, just a variant of normal? They can be very confident. When the pediatrician and cardiologist agree that a murmur is innocent, a heart problem is almost never found on additional tests. The trained ear is an excellent detective of innocent murmurs.

Several studies have been done to help physicians decide whether more or fewer children with murmurs should be seen by both a primary-care physician and a cardiologist. A recent study from Ottawa, published in the journal *Pediatrics* (October 1990) showed that pediatricians are good at detecting which children have mild defects rather than innocent murmurs. Most children with innocent murmurs are never referred to heart specialists. About 20 to 30 percent of all children with murmurs referred to specialists have innocent murmurs.

In case of doubt, an echo-Doppler study can aid in confirming normal function of the heart muscle and in making certain that no trivial defect or valve leakage is causing the murmur. An echo-Doppler test done expertly can detect extremely tiny, insignificant heart problems, even those hard to hear with a stethoscope. In Tommy's case all tests confirmed that he is a healthy boy with a normal heart and an innocent murmur. Tommy's family should not wait anxiously for him to "grow out of it"; he is normal *now*.

Does every child with a heart murmur need an echo-Doppler test?

This is a tough question, for as we said at the outset each child is unique and a decision must be based on individual circumstances. For example, if a murmur is heard in infancy in an otherwise healthy baby and is still heard at 2 years of age, a cardiologist's opinion will often be requested. The echo-Doppler test can be a useful supplement to a cardiologist's physical examination; however, the echocardiogram should be interpreted as *part* of a complete examination. In an older child, the pediatrician is often confident that a murmur is innocent, and tests confirm this opinion 95 percent of the time. If the physician is uncertain, a pediatric cardiology consultation is often requested.

Will Tommy ever become really active in sports?

Tommy's uncle once played lacrosse for the Hopkins Blue Jays, so the family is intensely interested in this question. The answer has nothing to do with Tommy's innocent heart murmur. His athletic potential lies in that combination of genes, muscle coordination, speed, and motivation that distinguishes the accomplished athlete from the rest of us. His innocent heart murmur is irrelevant to the question. We have often found that parents can accept the idea that the murmur will not stop a child, while the grandparents remain anxious. "Can he really play Little League now he has this heart murmur?" they may ask. Reading the American Heart Association's booklets about innocent heart murmurs can help the family share in understanding the normal, healthy, fully active future that lies ahead. Also, the grandparents' own physician can help by emphasizing the great reliability of modern methods of diagnosis and the value of exercise and full activity in the continuing heart health of children and adults alike.

Fortunately, Tommy's family shared their thoughts with each other, and their joy in Tommy and in his activities grew as he did.

Innocent heart murmurs need not be followed in a heart clinic. If something changes, the pediatrician can always arrange for a repeat check, but this will hardly ever be necessary.

Not all murmurs *are* innocent. Some are a sign of problems, some mild, some not. These are discussed in the chapters that follow.

Benign Mitral Valve Prolapse

Verne went for a physical examination before starting to play on her school's girls' hockey team at age 12. She was very athletic, and no heart problem had ever been detected. The pediatrician noted that Verne's heart sounded normal while she was lying down, but that when she sat up or stood up, an extra clicking sound could be heard. He sent her to the cardiologist, who confirmed this finding and asked for an echo test. The echo showed that the posterior leaflet of the mitral valve bowed upward (prolapsed) into the left atrium with each heartbeat, but that there was no leakage or insufficiency of the mitral valve. Verne and her par-

ents were advised that she could play on the hockey team and that she did not require any medication. A follow-up visit in about five years' time was recommended to make sure the prolapse had not progressed as she grew, as does occur in a few teenagers. When she was reexamined at 18 years, before going to college, the clicking sound and the echo test were unchanged.

Tracy E. was at a baseball game with her parents and her younger brother. The Orioles were winning. Suddenly Mr. E. asked his wife if she heard a loud noise, almost like the honking of a goose. It seemed to come from Tracy's chest. Tracy felt fine, but her parents were naturally somewhat anxious, and her 10-year-old brother found the noise embarrassing! After talking with the pediatrician by phone, the family came to the heart center. When the E's were told that a mitral valve prolapse sometimes showed itself in this way, Mr. E. said that he had been told that he had mitral valve prolapse a year ago, after a doctor noticed a click in his own chest. Tracy's honking sound faded over the next few days, and although she continues to have mitral valve prolapse, it has never "acted up" like that again. Both she and her father take BE prophylaxis but are otherwise perfectly healthy.

The word *prolapse* implies displacement; in benign mitral valve prolapse, the two leaflets of the mitral valve do not meet perfectly when the heart beats. Instead, one or both leaflets, usually the posterior one, is out of place and produces a clicking sound as it moves. It is difficult to say definitely how many children have MVP, but we can say that MVP in children is almost always benign (probably 95 percent of the time). Prolapse is found in only about 1 percent of babies, but the incidence increases to 3 to 5 percent in 10-year-olds. Billowing or scalloping of the mitral valve leaflets (figure 9.2) is common and is now thought of as a normal variant. In a small minority, MVP is associated with moderate or severe mitral insufficiency and needs careful follow-up and treatment (see chapter 11).

Increasingly, cardiologists are emphasizing that prolapse without any thickening of the mitral valve leaflets or mitral insufficiency is a "nondisease," certainly during childhood. Many children and young adults may have a click: some will have MVP diagnosed on echo but not clinically. Most of these young people are being "delabelled," and the concept of normal variation of the mitral valve is being emphasized.

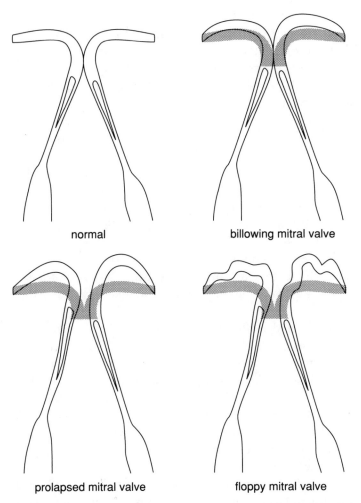

normal

billowing mitral valve

prolapsed mitral valve

floppy mitral valve

9.2. Mitral Valve Abnormalities. In the normal mitral valve, both leaflets meet smoothly when the ventricle beats and the valve closes; each leaflet is attached to the heart muscle by delicate chordae (cords). In *billowing mitral valve*, the leaflets are scalloped or irregular but function well. In true *prolapse*, one or both leaflets move upward into the left atrium; sometimes, as shown here, the leaflets do not close completely, resulting in some leakage backward from the left ventricle to the left atrium. (This condition is mitral valve prolapse with mitral insufficiency.) In *floppy mitral valve*, a rare form of mitral valve abnormality usually seen only in Marfan and a few other syndromes, the leaflets are floppy and redundant and the chordae supporting the leaflets may also be longer than normal and irregular. In this abnormality, significant mitral valve leakage or insufficiency is common and often progresses as the child grows.

In MVP, as in a number of other heart problems, there is a spectrum of severity; at one end of the spectrum, a trivial variation in the normal smooth geometry of the mitral valve, at the other end, a progressive and difficult problem that may need surgery. Some people with MVP have a complex of symptoms—including irregular heart rhythms, sweating, nervousness, and even panic attacks—referred to as *MVP syndrome* (see chapter 11). In this chapter we consider the trivial (benign) variation of MVP that is, in effect, normal and is of no medical concern.

The mitral valve, which lies between the left atrium and left ventricle of the heart, has two leaflets that normally meet smoothly with each heartbeat. But sometimes one or both leaflets have a minor variation in geometry, resulting in some waviness or "scalloping" of the normally smooth leaflet surface. This variation, often called *billowing mitral valve*, is extremely common—about 5 in 100 teenagers and young adults have it. It does not progress or cause any symptoms and may be thought of as an intriguing variation in anatomy rather than an abnormality.

As the affected leaflet (usually the posterior leaflet of the mitral valve) prolapses (is displaced upward), some blood may leak back into the left atrium with every heartbeat. The mitral valve, because it is allowing blood to leak backwards into the atrium, is then said to be "insufficient." When the insufficiency is trivial, as it usually is, a soft murmur may be heard, but sometimes the leak can be detected only with the echo-Doppler study. In some children who have mild degrees of prolapse, a soft heart murmur may be heard sometimes, but not always. Before the days when echo-Doppler testing was available, this intermittent nature of the murmur was a cause of controversy, and parents were baffled by the differing opinions of different doctors. Nowadays, a good Doppler study can show conclusively whether or not there is MVP, whether mitral insufficiency is present, and—if it is—whether it is trivial.

MVP is more common in girls than in boys, and in people who are tall and slender rather than short and stocky. MVP is most common in healthy teenagers and young adults. It often runs in families, from one generation to another. When it does so, geneticists say it is inherited as an *autosomal dominant with varying penetrance*; that is, if a mother or father has MVP there is a 40- to 50-percent chance that their child will also have it, but the time of appearance of the click and the degree of prolapse varies a great deal inside any given family.

How does mild MVP affect the child?

It doesn't. There is now agreement that in its mild form MVP is so frequent as to be a normal variant that can safely be ignored. It should not be considered for insurance purposes, or in giving advice regarding activity. In a severe form, surgery for MVP *is* necessary, although it is almost never needed except in children with Marfan syndrome. The rare form of severe progressive MVP is usually seen only in children with Marfan syndrome or some other connective tissue disorder that affects many different parts of the body. Surgery on the mitral valve may be necessary in a few such children.

Benign mitral valve prolapse is detected when the physician listening to the heart hears a clicking sound (this sound is loud enough for a parent to hear in fewer than one child in several thousand), heard especially easily when the child is sitting or standing, not lying down. It is quite common and is a benign variant of normal. An echo-Doppler test is often recommended to confirm that there is no other problem in the heart. When there is none, no cardiac follow-up is needed, and the child can live normally.

Very occasionally, a child or adult who has MVP intermittently develops a loud honking murmur that can be heard even without a stethoscope. This was the sound Tracy's family heard. This intermittent honking murmur was described almost 100 years ago, before the first diagnosis of MVP. It is thought that one of the chordae (cords) supporting the valve leaflets alters its shape or position temporarily, so that blood coursing through the ventricle makes it twang or vibrate in this unusual way. The honking happens in only a tiny minority of MVP patients and has no ill effects.

Mitral insufficiency causes a heart murmur, which is usually very soft when the problem is mild. Children with mild mitral insufficiency are usually advised to have a follow-up cardiac examination and echo-Doppler every two to five years, and antibiotic coverage (BE prophylaxis) is advised for dental work and similar procedures to avoid any risk of bacterial infection of the mitral valve, or bacterial endocarditis (see chapter 14).

In summary, it is not unusual for a murmur to be heard in a child whose heart was thought to be normal in infancy, but the overwhelming majority of such murmurs are innocent and require no treatment or follow-up. When the murmur is caused by a mild congenital heart defect, the defect itself is not treated, but antibiotic coverage to prevent endocarditis is advised: for example, a child who has a small ventricular septal defect will need to have antibiotics before any dental work is done, until the defect has closed completely and the murmur has gone.

Children with benign MVP lead normal lives and are fully active; they need preventive measures against endocarditis only when the mitral valve is thickened or abnormal, or if mitral insufficiency is complicating the prolapse.

Thus, although the children discussed in this chapter are healthy and active and need no medication or surgery for their hearts, some of them do need BE prophylaxis before they have dental work or other operations and others do not. The American Heart Association recommends the following for children with the problems discussed in this chapter: no treatment and no prophylaxis for anyone with innocent murmurs or benign MVP (without any thickening of the mitral valve leaflets or mitral insufficiency), or with a bicuspid pulmonary valve. Those children who do need BE prophylaxis are all other children who have congenital heart defects, however mild, including those with small ventricular septal defects (until that defect has closed). Prophylaxis is particularly important for children who have aortic valve problems, including those with a bicuspid aortic valve. Children with mitral valve prolapse with thickened valve leaflets or with mitral insufficiency should also receive prophylaxis.

Chapter 10

Problems That Require Emergency Treatment after Birth

Some of the greatest advances in treatment of children's heart problems have occurred in the management of the most severe, that is, *critical*, heart defects. We use the term critical to mean that a severe defect in a newborn infant needs urgent treatment. Some such defects can now be treated early with impressive success. Until the mid-1960s, for example, an infant born with transposition had less than a 5-percent chance of reaching the first birthday, but, successful surgery for transposition can usually be done in the first week of life. The baby with transposition, who once would have lived only briefly and precariously, is lively and healthy.

The initial diagnosis of a heart problem, especially a critical one, provokes intense anxiety and many questions. After urgent treatment of a newborn has begun, new questions will arise—less urgent, perhaps, but still pressing. Parents' questions may focus on the best resource for treatment: Should their child be treated by the local cardiology team, for example, or be transferred to a medical "Mecca," a heart center frequently in the news for its pioneering work? They face what is often a terrifying dilemma. They may have been unaware that a child could be born with a heart defect at all; now they learn that their baby, so long awaited and so helpless, requires immediate heart surgery to survive. What questions should they ask? How can they know that the doctor talking to them, a cardiologist who may be younger than they, really is expert enough to deal with their child's heart problem and their own anxieties?

Fortunately, there has been great progress in achieving high standards for the care of children's hearts. Almost all large children's hospitals have on their staffs cardiologists who are fully trained in pediatrics, with three or more years' training in pediatric cardiology at a major university before their certification. It is often helpful for parents to talk to the pediatrician about his or her experience with the cardiac care team and to ask for help in understanding the options available. Most of the time families can be confident that their local heart center can, indeed, offer competent skilled care and that there is no need to travel far from home. Most major children's heart centers now handle newborn emergencies well.

Fortunately, more and more babies who start life needing emergency treatment to correct a heart defect are able to go home within one or two weeks after birth, and many grow and develop just as they would if they had never been critically ill. Of all babies born with defects, that is about eight out of one thousand babies, three or four will need treatment before their first birthday, and two or three of these will have critical problems that require emergency treatment soon after birth.

Problems That May Cause a Critical Illness in a Newborn

Although occasionally a viral illness transmitted from the mother may cause a baby to be born with myocarditis (inflammation of the heart muscle) and heart failure, most critical heart problems are caused by a severe congenital defect; that is, the heart did not develop normally as the baby was growing in the womb. Some of these problems are recognized before birth, through fetal echocardiography. (When a fetal heart abnormality is detected during an ultrasound test, the mother is sent for special echo studies of the fetal heart.) Sometimes, then, an abnormal fetal heart rhythm or an illness of the mother may lead to diagnosis of a baby's heart defect before the baby is born.

In most pregnancies, however, there is no suspicion of a heart defect. Because the placenta supplies not only nutrition but oxygen to the growing fetus, a fetus that is not receiving a normal flow of blood from the heart to the lungs can continue to grow in the womb. But immediately after birth, with the baby's first cry, oxygen has to come from the baby's own lungs. For babies born with *cyanotic heart defects*, resulting in dangerously low oxygen levels in the body, emergency treatment is needed. Transposition and hypoplastic right ventricle are two causes of this type of problem.

When the arteries are transposed, or connected wrongly to the heart, blood returning from the body does not reach the lungs for a new supply of oxygen (see chapter 5). The baby becomes intensely blue (cyanotic) shortly after birth and needs urgent treatment. In other babies, the entire right side of the heart is too small. (In chapter 4 we discussed how defects can be caused by abnormal flow through the right side of the heart while the baby is in the womb.) In the most severe defects, the right ventricle is tiny and does not allow blood to reach the lungs in the usual way. The baby is born intensely blue and has dangerously low levels of oxygen in the arteries supplying the body.

In babies with a severe obstruction on the left side of the heart, oxygen can reach the lungs, but the baby may become acutely ill and short of breath within hours or days of birth. The baby has a severe left-heart flow defect. The obstruction from this defect may not cause a severe problem immediately, because the ductus is still open and acts as a kind of bypass. As soon as the ductus closes, however, the defect will need to be treated. Coarctation of the aorta, aortic valve stenosis, and hypoplastic left ventricle are all defects of this kind (these defects are discussed in chapter 4).

Sometimes *heart failure*, with congestion of the baby's lungs and body, occurs shortly after birth. There are a number of causes of such heart failure. In some babies there is a severe conotruncal defect, such as a truncus arteriosus (see chapter 5). In others a very complex heart problem, such as single ventricle with coarctation, may be the cause. In the most fortunate group, there is only one defect. Stephanie, a premature baby with a patent ductus arteriosus who is described in one of the stories that follow, was treated rapidly and successfully for newborn heart failure.

To summarize, critical heart problems requiring emergency care in the newborn period may be considered in three major groups:

1. Newborns with *cyanotic heart defects*, including transposition and hypoplastic right ventricle, may need urgent care; these babies are blue (cyanotic) because blood cannot reach the lungs to obtain needed oxygen.

2. Babies with *obstruction* of blood flow in the left side of the heart due to coarctation, interrupted aortic arch, severe aortic stenosis, or hypoplastic left ventricle may appear normal at birth but become acutely ill as the ductus closes. Many can be helped by emergency surgery.

3. Babies with *heart failure* (congestion of the lungs and the body) require immediate treatment. Some of these babies have a single defect, such as patent ductus, which can be readily treated. Others have more severe problems, such as truncus arteriosus or anomalous pulmonary veins. And some have several complex defects requiring multiple operations.

Cyanotic Heart Defects

The infants in the following stories were intensely blue after birth and required emergency treatment.

Transposition of the great arteries

Marcus C. was born following a completely normal pregnancy. He weighed seven pounds at birth and looked healthy except that he was blue. The tension of oxygen in his arterial blood (pO_2) was measured by inserting a tiny needle into his radial artery: the level was only 30 torr, whereas the normal level is between 70 and 120. The level did not rise at all after Marcus spent ten minutes in an oxygen hood. This very low pO_2 is close to the level of about twenty torr, which leads to complications and early death.

Marcus was so vigorous and cried so normally when he was born that his parents had a hard time believing he needed immediate transfer to a heart center. But he was cyanotic. He received a chest X-ray and electrocardiogram and was started on an intravenous drip containing prostaglandin E1 to keep his ductus open, so that as much blood as possible would reach his lungs for oxygenation. At the children's center, where he was sent for treatment of his heart, he was put in a newborn intensive care unit. Most of the babies there were frail, tiny premature babies; Marcus looked big and healthy beside them.

After echo-Doppler and other tests were performed, the cardiologist explained to Marcus's father that his son had transposition of the great arteries. He arranged a family conference for the next day, when Mrs. C. would be out of the hospital. In the meantime Mr. C. looked at the videotape of the echo-Doppler study and a drawing and booklet describing transposition. By the time of the conference, it was agreed that Marcus would have surgery in the next few days. No heart catheter test would be needed to confirm the diagnosis.

Marcus had open-heart surgery when he was 4 days old. His aorta and pulmonary artery (which were transposed at birth) were each cut across shortly after they left the heart and rejoined to supply a normal circulation. The coronary arteries were moved to the new aorta. By the end of the operation the oxygen tension in his arterial blood was 200, ten times what it had been at birth. He had a very good recovery and was home when he was 10 days old, feeding well and looking a healthy pink. He has continued to grow and develop like a normal baby in the five years since then.

Marcus had transposition of the arteries: he was blue because blood could not reach his lungs for oxygenation. In a conotruncal defect, the great arteries are wrongly connected to the heart: the aorta connects to the right ventricle instead of the left and the pulmonary artery connects to the left ventricle instead of the right (figure 10.1).

With transposition, cyanosis is seen very soon after birth and does not improve with the administration of oxygen. The baby may be completely normal otherwise, and except for the blue color it may seem that nothing is wrong. Nevertheless, speedy diagnosis and immediate treatment in a special cardiac center are critically important.

Most people who look at a diagram of transposition (figure 10.1) will think the logical answer is to surgically switch the arteries to their normal positions, so the aorta is connected to the left ventricle as it should be and the pulmonary artery is connected to the right ventricle (figure 10.1). Such an *arterial switch*, or Jatene operation, was done for Marcus.

After the arterial switch most babies appear quite normal. Because the technique is relatively new, however, infants who have had an arterial switch have not been followed for a long enough period to be sure the arteries will grow properly where they have been switched. We do know that occasionally the artery, usually the "new" pulmonary artery, becomes narrowed at the place of switching, and that a further operation will be necessary. Therefore, at least twice in the first year after surgery and then every one or two years, follow-up echo-Doppler tests are needed to view these areas clearly.

The change in outlook for an infant born with transposition is quite dramatic; only thirty years ago virtually all infants like Marcus died in early infancy. Now Marcus is in kindergarten, looking healthy in every way and keeping up with his playmates.

For many years before the arterial switch (the surgery Marcus had)

A.

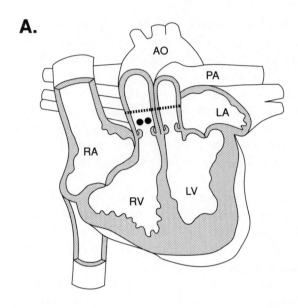

B.

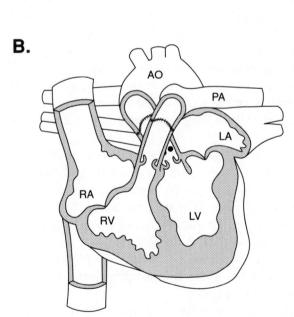

10.1. Arterial Switch for Transposition. *A,* In transposition the aorta (*AO*) is connected to the right ventricle (*RV*), the pulmonary artery (*PA*) to the left ventricle (*LV*). At the arterial switch (Jatene) procedure, the coronary arteries (their openings are shown as *black dots* in the aorta) are moved, each with a cuff of tissue around it. The aorta and pulmonary artery are both divided (shown by *dotted line*). *B,* Each artery is now reconnected to the appropriate ventricle; each coronary artery and surrounding cuff of tissue is sewn into the new aorta.

became available, other operations for transposition were used, because too many technical difficulties were involved in moving the coronary arteries over the new aorta. *Atrial switch* operations, such as the Mustard and the Senning operations, were developed in the mid-1960s and continue to be preferred over the arterial switch by some centers. Children who have had a Mustard operation or other kind of atrial switch have been observed for a much longer time than have children treated by an arterial switch.

In both the Mustard and Senning operations, blood is rerouted in the atrium; blue venous blood is directed to the left ventricle and from there it reaches the lungs. Blood from the lungs, containing normal levels of oxygen, passes behind the new piece of material ("baffle") in the atrium to the tricuspid valve, the right ventricle, and then to the aorta (figure 10.2). The atrial switch is one of the few times when two wrongs make a right! Now that the venous blood can obtain oxygen the baby is no longer cyanotic. For 20 years, from the mid-1960s to the mid-1980s, most infants with transposition underwent two or three procedures, in the following sequence:

1. As soon as the diagnosis of transposition was suspected, the baby was taken to the cardiac catheterization laboratory. There the foramen ovale, the small defect in the atrial septum normally present at birth, was enlarged with a balloon catheter (figure 10.3). This *Rashkind balloon atrial septostomy* was a wonderful advance, allowing infants to live who previously would have died.

2. Between two and twelve months later another catheterization was performed to check on the level of pressure in the pulmonary artery and to make certain that an atrial switch was feasible.

3. An atrial switch—Mustard or Senning operation—was performed shortly thereafter.

A Rashkind balloon atrial septostomy (figure 10.3), followed later by an atrial switch, is still used in a number of centers, often with excellent outcome. Fortunately, it is now feasible to do the atrial switch earlier than in past years, with less risk of complications from lower than normal oxygen levels in the blood.

Jimmy M., who is now 23 years old, was born with transposition and a ventricular septal defect. An atrial defect was created surgi-

A.

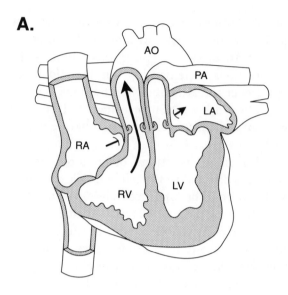

B.

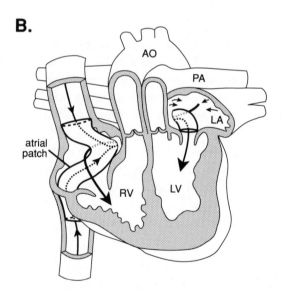

10.2. Mustard Atrial Switch for Transposition.

A, Before operation venous blood returning from the body enters the right atrium (*RA*) and then from the right ventricle (*RV*) to the aorta (*AO*), as shown by *large arrow.* Some blood passes between the right (*RA*) and left atrium (*LA*) as shown by *small arrow. B,* At operation the atrial septum is removed; a patch or baffle is placed in the atrium to direct blue venous blood from the right to the left atrium, then through the mitral valve to the left ventricle (*LV*) and pulmonary artery (*PA*) to reach the lungs. Blood containing oxygen returns via the pulmonary veins (shown as *four small arrows*) to the left atrium and then behind the baffle to the right atrium, right ventricle, and aorta to reach the body. New blood flow channels are shown by *large arrows* in each ventricle.

A.

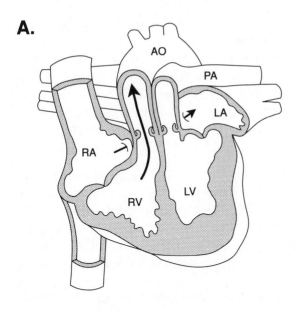

B.

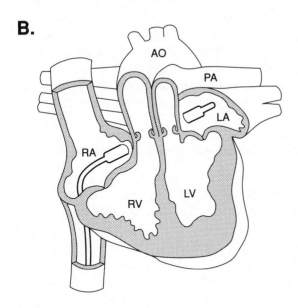

10.3. Rashkind Balloon Atrial Septostomy.
A, Before the septostomy, in a baby with transposition, blue venous blood returns from the body and passes into the right ventricle (*RV*) and aorta (*AO*), as shown by large arrow. [Oxygen-containing blood from the lungs enters the left atrium (*LA*), then the left ventricle (*LV*) and goes back to the lungs again via the pulmonary artery (*PA*)]. Once the ductus has closed, mixing of blood between the two circulations depends on the tiny foramen ovale, shown as a *small arrow* between the right (*RA*) and left atrium (*LA*). *B,* A balloon catheter is passed from a leg vein through the foramen ovale into the left atrium; the balloon is then inflated and pulled back across the atrial septum. This enlarges the atrial defect and allows more mixing of the circulations, so that some oxygen-containing blood from the lungs can reach the right atrium, right ventricle, and so reach the aorta and the body.

cally when he was 6 months old, to help relieve his blueness. At 3 years, he had a Mustard operation.

Jimmy finished high school and works full time as a mechanic. He and his wife are expecting their first baby shortly. Although he has felt well, a pacemaker was placed in his heart last year because he had a very slow, irregular heart rate, which had been present since his surgery and was gradually getting worse.

Jimmy is a gallant young man who exemplifies the pioneer patient who has grown as heart surgery has grown. His heart rhythm is now well controlled by a pacemaker. He needs careful follow-up for the pacemaker, and also to see whether the right ventricle can tolerate the high pressure needed to supply the aorta over a normal life span. So far his right ventricle, although much larger than normal, has done very well.

Major variants of transposition include additional heart defects; the most usual among the extra defects are large ventricular septal defects, pulmonary stenosis, and abnormalities of the mitral or tricuspid valves. Occasionally the baby is premature or has a complicated syndrome, and such babies almost always have a more prolonged and difficult course. Occasionally repair of the heart will not be possible, and the baby will not survive. Marcus was born with the usual kind of transposition; he had no other defects in his heart or body. Some people call this "simple transposition," although it is not a simple defect for the family or surgeon.

Hypoplastic right ventricle with pulmonary atresia

Amanda Q. was blue immediately after birth, even though she was a full-term vigorous baby and had a good loud cry. The nursery where she was born was an excellent one, but after Amanda had had an X-ray and an electrocardiogram, her parents were told that she would need to be transferred to a nursery with special cardiac facilities. She had a hypoplastic right ventricle, a serious defect. She was started on a prostaglandin E1 infusion, and her color improved.

Amanda experienced no trouble during the ride in the ambulance, but soon after arriving in the new neonatal intensive care unit she suddenly stopped breathing. She revived quickly, and her dose of prostaglandin was reduced, because prostaglandins can sometimes cause sudden episodes of breathing failure. Echo-Doppler and other tests confirmed that Amanda had a tiny right ventricle and atresia of the pulmonary valve. After a cardiac catheterization study it was recommended that she have an operation to open her pulmonary valve and to perform a Blalock-Taussig shunt.

Amanda went home with her parents a week after surgery, off medications and doing well, although her color remained a little blue. Her pulmonary valve and right ventricle remained tiny, and at 6 months she had another catheter test. A balloon catheter opened up her pulmonary valve a little more, but not enough to make the ventricle grow.

At 7 months Amanda had a second operation to remove some of the thick muscle in her right ventricle and to put a patch on the front wall of the ventricle to give it a bigger cavity. Again she did well, and she went home eight days later. When she was 2 years of age her right ventricle was almost normal size; she had a third operation to put in a pulmonary valve and to close the defect in her atrial septum and close off the shunt. Now 8 years old, Amanda is doing well in school and needs no medications. She is checked once a year in the heart clinic.

In a child with a hypoplastic right ventricle, the right ventricle, which should be pumping blood to the lungs, is a tiny muscle-bound slit and cannot pump efficiently (figure 4.4). In an infant like Amanda, the pulmonary valve is completely closed (this is pulmonary atresia), so although blood can enter the right ventricle during the time the heart is developing, it has nowhere to go. The right ventricle is a blind cavity that has thick walls but sends no blood to the lungs. The tricuspid valve is present but is very small.

While Amanda was in the womb there was no sign of difficulty. Oxygen was provided by the placenta. But soon after birth she became cyanotic. She was started on an intravenous dose of prostaglandin E1 to keep the ductus open while plans were being developed for her transfer and treatment. (If the pulmonary valve is sealed shut, blood flow to the lungs must depend entirely on the ductus, and if the ductus closes, the infant cannot survive. For this reason hypoplastic right ventricle is a cardiac emergency.) Very often the neonatologist or doctor referring a baby like Amanda will already have obtained test results that point toward the hypoplastic right ventricle—for example, an EKG may show the left ventricle to be the dominant one, which is an abnormal condition immediately after birth. The shape of the heart on a chest X-ray may also be helpful, since the shape indicates that the right ventricle is small. An echo-Doppler test will show the closed-off valve or valves and the tiny right ventricle, and will indicate whether any blood is reaching the lungs directly from the heart or whether everything depends on the ductus. Because the treatment of such cases is so difficult, cardiac catheterization will often be done quickly after the baby is first seen, to help define a treatment plan.

It is almost impossible to give a summary of all the possible treatment plans for the severe condition of hypoplastic right ventricle. Often doctors try to paint an optimistic picture by talking about methods of improving blood flow to the lungs. There are many such methods, many of them good, but the small right ventricle is the crux of the problem, and it is difficult to treat.

Amanda is a joy to her family and is a great example of successful modern procedures applied to what was once an almost hopeless heart problem. By 3 years of age she had had three cardiac catheterizations and three operations, more than most people need in their whole lives. She was fortunate that her right ventricle, although small, was capable of some growth once blood was flowing through it after her birth. This is not always the case. In every child with pulmonary atresia the aim is to increase blood flow to the lungs as an emergency short-term measure, and to help the right ventricle grow so that eventually an almost normal circulation is achieved.

Amanda's successful outcome is an inspiration, but there is no quick fix for a small right ventricle. Her parents not only had to undergo the ordeal of spending many days and nights in the hospital, but they had to sign many consent forms full of explicit details of all the dire complications that might possibly occur at each procedure. Like many other young parents of a sick child, they found that their friends and contemporaries, while friendly and sympathetic, really had no concept or understanding of life with constant illness. Fortunately, their devotion to each other and to Amanda and her younger brother has grown deeper with time.

Both Marcus and Amanda had cyanotic defects and dangerously low oxygen levels in their blood. The next two stories describe John P. and Zachary G., both of whom also had emergency heart surgery as newborns but whose problem was not lack of oxygen. In both boys the connection between the right ventricle and the lungs was normal, and in both boys the flow of blood to the body was inadequate. Each became acutely ill soon after birth because of a severe obstruction to the left side of the heart.

Obstruction of Blood Flow in the Left Side of the Heart

Coarctation of the aorta

John P. was a long-awaited baby whose parents had tried for several years to start a family and were seriously thinking of adoption before Mrs. P. became pregnant. All went well during the pregnancy, and John was born in a community hospital. He weighed seven pounds, two ounces, he was vigorous and healthy looking, and he breast-fed eagerly. At 3 days old he was about to go home with his mother when a nurse noticed that he was breathing fast. His discharge was delayed, and all the data, including his blood pressures, were rechecked. The pressure in his right arm was 80 mm Hg; the pressure in his legs only 50 mm Hg. A chest X-ray showed some enlargement of the heart; an EKG was normal. The pediatrician talked to the parents and arrangements were made for John to be seen at the nearby heart center on his way home. However, while the phone calls were being made, John began to breathe harder and to look pale and ill. He was started on prostaglandin E1 by intravenous infusion and transferred to the heart center, where the diagnosis of coarctation was confirmed by an echo-Doppler test. He also was found to have a bicuspid aortic valve, although the inside of his heart was normal and the ventricle was pumping well.

John went to surgery the next day. The left subclavian artery was used to enlarge the narrowed area, and the ductus was divided. He needed some medication in the pediatric intensive care unit to lower his blood pressure, but otherwise he did well.

John went home with his parents five days after the operation and breast-fed well. He was a happy, lively baby. At his 6-month checkup he showed signs of restenosis; the blood pressure in his arm was again higher than that in his leg, although he appeared well. The cardiologist recommended balloon dilation of the narrow area, and John went to the same-day care center and then to the catheterization laboratory. A balloon catheter was passed up from the femoral artery in his leg; after the balloon was inflated the obstruction was relieved. John was kept overnight in the intensive

care unit to be sure that no sudden changes in blood pressure occurred, but the night passed uneventfully. John has remained entirely well and has regular checkups with his pediatrician. He is
seen in the heart center once a year.

*Why did John have this problem? Was it somehow related to his
parents' difficulty in conceiving? Or to some medication exposure
of his parents at work? Or was there some other reason?*

No studies to date have shown that difficulty in conception or frequent prior miscarriages are risk factors for coarctation or other left-
heart flow defects (see chapter 3 for a discussion of risk factors). Nor
have any medications proven to be a cause of such defects. In the BWIS
there was some suggestion that parental exposure to industrial solvents
is a minor risk factor, but this is far from proven. In any case, neither of
John's parents was exposed to solvents at work; John's mother was a
secretary, his father an accountant, and neither had any hobbies involving the use of solvents. Because both parents were extremely interested
in understanding more about John's problem, they volunteered for a
family study. Mr. P. himself was found to have a bicuspid aortic valve,
suggesting some genetic predisposition. The pregnancy factors that
may influence expression of this genetic predisposition are now under
study.

The principle of treatment of coarctation of the aorta (figure 4.5) is
to relieve the obstruction in the aorta and eliminate the shelf blocking
the free flow of blood from the upper to the lower body by opening the
left side of the chest and repairing the aorta. The heart-lung machine is
not needed.

In the early years of heart surgery the aorta was clamped above and
below the coarctation, the narrowed segment was removed, and the
two cut ends were sewn back together. This resection with end-to-end
anastomosis (cutting out and joining together) was a satisfactory operation for older children and adults. Some surgeons now use a combination of methods in babies. Preliminary follow-up studies of children
who have been operated on in infancy or early childhood suggest that
their left ventricles are much healthier than the left ventricles of patients who had surgery later in life.

Will the coarctation recur a third time? Or keep on coming back?

Because balloon dilation has been done for only a few years, we do not
yet know for certain how long it will be effective. However, all the

older studies on reoperation for coarctation suggest that the chance of a third recurrence is extremely low, less than one in one thousand, particularly in view of the fact that John's balloon dilation was so successful in relieving the obstruction. A few children who have had this procedure done show some thinning of the aortic wall where the balloon has been inflated. John's parents understood that this had not happened to their child, but they also realized that it would help John and other children if he continued to be seen by the cardiac team so that any possible complications could be recognized and treated immediately.

Hypoplastic left ventricle with aortic atresia

Zachary G. had grown rather slowly in the middle part of his mother's pregnancy. A fetal ultrasound test at twenty-eight weeks showed a small left ventricle and a very tiny aorta. His parents were told that the doctors suspected their baby had aortic atresia with hypoplastic left ventricle. After much discussion Mrs. G. elected to arrange for delivery in a nearby city where there was a cardiac surgical team specializing in the Norwood operation.

Zachary was born at 38 weeks weighing six pounds. He was seen immediately after birth by the cardiologist and the diagnosis was confirmed. He remained on prostaglandins for two days while tests were being done to make sure he had no other problems. When he was 4 days old he underwent heart surgery. He remained in the intensive care unit for seven days but was discharged home with his parents at 18 days old. He returned for a second operation when he was 7 months old.

When he was almost 3 years old and small for his age but developing normally, Zachary had his third operation. That procedure was successful, and he will need no more surgery. He is now 5 and still doing well.

When the left ventricle fails to grow normally, the right ventricle maintains the circulation during life in the womb. Before birth Zachary grew a little slowly but otherwise, as is usual, there was no difficulty. His problem was discovered by fetal echocardiography at twenty-eight weeks' gestation, and arrangements were made for him to be delivered in a center with facilities for treatment immediately after birth. Zachary was lucky. Most such babies are born with no one suspecting that they have a serious heart defect.

Prostaglandins were started immediately so the ductus would stay open while various options for treatment were considered. Without prostaglandins, death usually ensues within a few hours or days. Of all infants in the BWIS region who were born between 1981 and 1985 with hearts like Zachary's, only 10 in 100 lived to see their first birthday. Each year more infants do well, but hypoplastic left ventricle with aortic atresia (figure 4.5) is still a serious problem and several operations are required.

The operation Zachary had, the *Norwood procedure*, is a complicated one. It involves joining the tiny aorta to the large pulmonary artery to make a single vessel to supply both the body and the lungs. It is a very delicate and difficult operation but can now be done successfully about seven times out of ten, though only in certain centers. In the second stage of the operation, which is usually not done before 2 years of age, the entire circulation is made to bypass the tiny left ventricle. In Zachary's case this operation was done at 7 months. It is a variant of the Fontan operation used for children with hypoplastic right ventricle (see chapter 13). In some children surgeons are now doing an intermediate procedure, joining the caval veins to the pulmonary artery, at the end of the first year of life; the Fontan operation is postponed until the child is 3 years old or older.

Dr. Leonard Bailey of Loma Linda, California, was the first surgeon to perform a heart transplant for this condition. More than forty such transplants have been done worldwide, and about eight of ten of these babies have lived for one or more years after transplant. The uncertainty about having a donor heart available soon enough and the need for very close postoperative supervision to prevent rejection of the new heart have made this a controversial technique; it is available only in a few heart centers.

Many families presented with the difficult choice outlined here feel that no therapy should be started other than compassionate supportive care. Whatever the decision and however strong and supportive the family constellation, this is an agonizing time for the parents. One must hope that in future years more infants will have Zachary's good outcome, and that ultimately we will learn how to prevent this tragic disorder.

Until very recently hypoplastic left ventricle was uniformly fatal by age 3 months, and most babies died before they were 1 week old. Even now only a few cardiac centers have had any consistent success with surgery. The right approach remains a subject of debate.

Heart Failure in Newborns with Enlargement of the Heart and Congestion of the Lungs

The next two stories describe babies who developed heart failure with enlargement of the heart and congestion of the lungs while they were still in the newborn nursery.

Patent ductus arteriosus causing heart failure in a premature baby

Stephanie was born at 28 weeks (twelve weeks prematurely) weighing only one pound, five ounces. She was vigorous, but her lungs were immature and she needed extra oxygen for several days. Just as her lungs began to look better on her chest X-ray, she developed a loud murmur over her chest and again began to need more oxygen. Her heart was enlarged and overactive. The neonatalogist thought her murmur was due to a patent ductus; this diagnosis was confirmed by echo-Doppler testing, which showed a very large ductus. Stephanie was given less fluid than before and was also given indomethacin, a medication often useful in making the ductus close in premature babies. However, the ductus did not close.

Stephanie went to surgery at 9 days of age, still weighing only as much as she did at birth. An opening was made in the left side of her chest between the ribs, and the surgeon put some ligature around the ductus and then divided it. Like all other operations on the ductus, this was a closed-heart operation, meaning that the heart itself did not have to be opened, and so the heart-lung machine was not needed. Stephanie was back in the neonatal care unit less than an hour after being taken to the operating room. She improved quickly after the operation and oxygen was discontinued a few days later. Her heart returned to normal size and she never developed any other heart problems. She went home when she was 13 weeks old, weighing 4.5 pounds.

About one in three babies who weigh less than 1,500 grams at birth, as Stephanie did, need either medical or surgical treatment before the duct will close. The outcome is very good as far as the heart is concerned, although babies who are born prematurely may have many other problems related to their small size and the immaturity of their lungs. The ductus is part of the large public health problem of prematurity and low birth weight.

Patent ductus arteriosus, Stephanie's defect, is a continuation after birth of the channel that joins the aorta and the pulmonary artery. At birth the muscle in the wall of the ductus constricts, in response to the new higher level of oxygen in the blood, and blood stops passing through the ductus a few hours later. But the ductus may remain in a small premature infant like Stephanie in whom the muscle in the ductus wall is not yet mature enough to react to changes in oxygen. (In many premature infants the ductus will close after administration of the drug indomethacin, as discussed in chapter 4, and no further treatment is needed.) In a much smaller group of infants, the ductus muscle is defective even though the infant is born at full term.

Because the flow of blood in patent ductus, as in atrial and ventricular septal defects, is from the left side of the heart to the right, too much blood flows into the lungs; the larger the defect, the more excessive the flow. Stephanie's ductus was very large, and she required early and urgent treatment. In full-term babies who are not in heart failure, surgical repair is often done after the child is 1 year old.

In addition to surgery, a new device to close the ductus through a catheter approach is now being tested in a few centers. Studies to date look promising, although the device cannot be used in very small babies.

Persistent truncus arteriosus in a newborn infant

Shauna Z. was born in a small town on the Eastern Shore of Maryland. Immediately after birth the pediatrician noticed that her heart was very active and a loud heart murmur could be heard over her chest. She was not cyanotic. For the first two days she seemed vigorous but always breathed faster than normal. By the time she was 3 days old her liver had begun to enlarge, however, and her parents were told that Shauna had signs of heart failure and required immediate treatment. She had a chest X-ray, an EKG, and an echo-Doppler test. These tests confirmed that both her right and left ventricles were greatly enlarged; on an echocardiogram, only one large artery could be seen leaving her heart.

Shauna was started on a diuretic medication to relieve the congestion in her lungs and was transferred immediately to a university heart center. Her father and aunt travelled to the heart center; Mrs. Z. had undergone a cesarean section and had to remain at the local hospital. She had to participate by telephone with members of the cardiology health team in the decision for Shauna to undergo cardiac catheterization, and she found the cardiac nurse specialist particularly helpful in supplying details of what was going on. Shauna's pediatrician came to visit Mrs. Z. in the maternity ward and showed her, with the help of the American Heart Association booklet and diagrams, what was meant by a truncus arteriosus (figure 5.4) and how the surgeons would repair it. Fortunately, Shauna showed some improvement on medication and her mother was well enough to travel to the center before surgery was done. Mr. and Mrs. Z. were able to go over the details of the planned operation with the surgeon, Dr. Bruce Reitz, and other members of the cardiac team. They knew it was a complicated procedure: the ventricular septal defect had to be closed with a patch, and Shauna's pulmonary arteries had to be removed from her aorta and joined to the right ventricle with a special form of graft called a homograft.

Shauna had a very stormy time for a week after surgery, but she slowly recovered. She finally went home at 7 weeks of age, never having left the hospital before. Her parents were helped through the long and anxious time of waiting by the health team. The daily crises were discussed openly and yet gently. Perhaps no one except the surgeon played a greater role than the nurses, who helped Mrs. Z. keep her supply of breast milk flowing until Shauna was finally strong enough to feed from her mother's breast. Arrangements were made for the family to stay in a special low-cost parents' inn near the heart center, and as the hospital expenses mounted, health team members helped Mr. and Mrs. Z. with an application for assistance from the children's medical services program in their home state. Because Shauna needed life-saving surgery in infancy, her parents were able to obtain Social Security Disability Supplemental Income for her until her first birthday.

For Shauna and her family, the *triangle of understanding* described in the Introduction worked well. Shauna's pediatrician helped the family with all the early decisions, including advice on Shauna's transfer to a center with a staff skilled and experienced in the operation she needed; he also made the agonizing time of waiting easier than it might have been.

Shauna's parents had to consider a question of even greater urgency than where to go. "What are her chances?" This is an emotional and terrifying question to have to ask about a newborn child. On the one hand, they had heard so much about the wonders of modern medicine that they expected a perfect result from surgery; on the other hand, the fact that Shauna could have no voice in any decisions, and that they had to choose for her, filled them with dread. The diagnosis was helpful: the parents knew that without surgery Shauna had no chance at all. Other parents have to face decisions about operations that are matters of choice, not necessity, and find even these decisions very hard. The health team, from its experience of similar operations performed over the past five years, was able to tell Shauna's parents that she had a 90-percent chance of surviving surgery for her truncus arteriosus (figure 5.4) and about an 80- to 85-percent chance of avoiding any major postoperative complication. Of every twenty infants who undergo Shauna's particular operation, one will die and two will have major complications (see chapter 14). These figures are good—indeed, miraculous—when you remember that heart surgery began only in the 1940s. Yet, although it is important to know the statistics, Shauna is more than a heart defect and more than a statistic. Statistics apply to populations of patients, not to an individual. Shauna, like every other baby who undergoes heart surgery, will either live or die: it is these two absolutes, not percentages, that matter to her family.

Two years after the operation, when Shauna and her family went back to the heart center for a "cardiac birthday party," someone asked Mrs. Z., "What was the worst part? Was it waiting for her to come back from the operation? Or when you first knew she was not a healthy baby, as you had hoped?"

Mrs. Z. answered, "No. The worst moment was when someone said they had to cut into her heart. She was so tiny, so helpless, and to Dick and me, her heart was so precious. How could anyone cut into it? It made me sick even to think of it."

"How did you decide to let her have surgery?"

"I don't know. Dick and I came to the hospital one night, when visiting hours were almost over, and sat watching her under her oxygen hood. She was so beautiful, but she was so frail, and she was breathing so hard, even though she was asleep. Dick said to me, 'We both know she won't make it. We don't have any choice, do we?' I always think it was Shauna who showed us what to do, although we surely had a lot of help."

Although the defect Shauna had—truncus arteriosus—is an abnormality of the conotruncal area of the heart (see chapter 5), it usually shows itself by causing heart failure rather than cyanosis. Some such babies have Di George syndrome; that is, they have additional problems, such as low levels of calcium in the blood. Shauna was fortunate in having a defect involving only her heart.

Follow-up after Treatment

When Shauna returned home after her heart operation her parents were at first very anxious; every time she coughed or cried they worried about whether she was in pain or going back into heart failure. They made many telephone calls and visits to the pediatrician in the first few weeks; he and they also had frequent contacts with the cardiologist and cardiac nurse specialist. Everyone—the family, the pediatrician, and all the health team—focused on Shauna—her needs, her future, and her best interests.

As their immediate anxieties grew less, and Shauna started smiling and growing, a new set of questions arose:

- What should we watch for?
- Does she need a special diet?
- How often will she have to come back for tests?
- What about the scar on her chest?
- Will she be able to have children?

The answers to such questions vary depending on the specific heart problem. In general, signs for these parents to watch for include irritability, feeding difficulty, and fever. Shauna went home breast-feeding well; she seemed a happy baby. Sometimes, however, a baby who has had a long and difficult course in the hospital goes home cranky and feeding poorly; the parents may become quite exhausted at home and may bring the baby back to the emergency room repeatedly for reassurance, sometimes seeing a succession of different doctors. A great deal of this uncertainty can be alleviated if a public health nurse visits the home for a few weeks after the baby's discharge to help with feeding and to advise the new parents on how to care for their baby.

Follow-up visits are usually recommended two to four weeks after discharge, and then six months and one year later. A baby like Shauna, who has had a major heart operation, will usually be seen at least once a year. Because she has had a valve placed in her heart to replace her own missing pulmonary valve, she may need further heart surgery when she is around 10 years old, so it is vital that she be seen regularly. Shauna's family became quite attached to the technicians in the heart station who performed the echo tests and the EKGs, and sometimes brought them flowers and cookies. Even Shauna eventually stopped crying when she saw them.

Like Shauna, most children with heart problems need no special diet. A few, especially those who require more than one operation or who have defects in other organs, grow very slowly and may need more than the usual number of calories, since many of the calories they take in are wasted by the extra work the heart has to do. A nutritionist can provide an individual diet plan, and special nursing instructions can help if tube feedings are necessary at home.

When the cardiac surgeon joined the cardiologist to see Shauna at her first checkup, he could tell from the family's expressions and from looking at Shauna that all had gone well at home. He listened to her heart and studied the echo test, and agreed with Mr. and Mrs. Z. that everything was progressing favorably. The scar looked more red and raised now than it would in a few weeks; if Shauna found it unsightly later, plastic surgery could be done, although few children do ask for such repair. The surgeon and the cardiologist explained to the parents the reasons why Shauna needed to be seen again at intervals. Mrs. Z. drew out of her pocketbook the diagram her pediatrician had given her of the operation, and the surgeon went over it with the parents. They told the pediatrician later how reassured they had been by the surgeon's calm and quiet approach, both before and after surgery.

The last question the Z's asked—Will Shauna be able to have children?—is more complicated than it sounds. They are asking themselves and the health team, Will Shauna grow up? And if she does, will she bear children? Even if they do not put it into words, they are asking themselves also: Will her children be normal? Will she have to go through what we have just endured?

In general, if a child has had an uncomplicated and early complete repair of a heart defect, the chances of the child's reaching adulthood are excellent. The type of operation Shauna had has been done successfully for fewer than twenty years, but now, having survived the operation well, she has 98 in 100 chances of growing to adulthood. As an adult, she should be able to tolerate a pregnancy well, although of course she will need a cardiac checkup before undertaking a pregnancy. If her own family and the family of her future spouse are free of heart defects or syndromes, she has a 90-percent chance of having a child of her own who has a normal heart (see chapter 3).

The Range of Problems Requiring Emergency Treatment

The stories of children described in this chapter provide a few examples of how infants with critical heart problems can often have successful treatment. Cyanosis, obstruction of blood flow to the body, and **congestive heart failure** are all signs that the baby's heart needs urgent help. Heart defects vary not only in severity, but also in complexity, and success is not always possible. Additional problems outside the heart may also make treatment more difficult and prolonged. Later in the book we will describe examples of children with complex heart defects, with multiple handicaps, and with treatment failures. In the next two chapters we describe some children who needed treatment but whose problems were milder than those in this chapter, so that medication or surgery could be postponed until after one month of age.

Chapter 11

Problems That
May Be Treated
without Surgery

A number of heart problems that require treatment are treated not by surgery but with medications or catheterization. New medications have had a great influence on the treatment of childhood heart problems. Diuretics, for example, have been helpful in treating infants and children who have excessive fluid in the lungs due to heart failure. Other medications have been able to control abnormal heart rhythms and manipulate abnormalities of blood pressure. The advent of prostaglandin E1 treatment in the early 1980s, a major advance for sick newborns, kept the ductus open in many critically ill babies while needed studies were being done and preparations were being made for surgery; indomethacin became available to close the ductus in premature babies, thus often avoiding the need for surgery in these infants altogether.

Another great breakthrough occurred in the catheterization laboratory. Before 1966 the cardiac catheter was useful in diagnosis but not as a direct source of treatment. Then, in 1966, Dr. William Rashkind of Philadelphia developed a balloon catheter that could be used to enlarge a tiny opening in the atrial septum and help infants born with transposition of the great arteries (see figure 10.3). In 1983, Dr. Jean Kan of Johns Hopkins in Baltimore employed a balloon catheter to open up the narrowed pulmonary valve in children who had pulmonary stenosis. This method, called *pulmonary valvuloplasty*, is now used all over the world; it is sometimes described by the rather forbidding term "interventional cardiology." (Radiologists prefer the term "interventional radiology.") With this method of treatment, surgery could be delayed or completely avoided, and the child could often be treated without needing to be in the hospital even for a single night. Other catheters have been developed with devices to close a patent ductus or an atrial septal defect, but their future role is uncertain.

Medications can be of great value in the control of symptoms and in the management of an acute change in the function of the heart. Medication may be the *only* treatment, or it may be used as a prelude to surgery. Often medications are given for a time after surgery, while the heart and body are adjusting to the new circulation. Medical and surgical methods are often used collaboratively in infants and children with severe heart problems. A baby with a large ventricular septal defect, for example, will be tried on furosemide (Lasix) to control heart failure while the physicians wait to see whether the defect gets smaller. If it does, medication is stopped; if it does not, the baby will have surgery, with furosemide for a month or two after surgery.

The three most common uses of heart medications are these:

1. In the treatment and control of heart failure, sometimes referred to as *congestion*; or congestive heart failure.

2. In the control of arrhythmias, or abnormal heart rhythms. Arrhythmias, especially abnormally fast rhythms (tachycardias) in babies, or prolonged repeated tachycardias at any age, may lead to heart failure. Not all arrhythmias need treatment, but when they occur in infants or children with heart muscle disorders such as cardiomyopathy, or in children who have had earlier heart surgery, treatment with medications is usually advised.

3. In newborns, to treat the ductus. In some babies prostaglandin E1 keeps the ductus open until heart surgery can be done. In premature babies, indomethacin may be used to close the ductus.

Medications for the Treatment and Control of Heart Failure

Jake L. had been born prematurely and weighed only 2.5 pounds at birth. He breathed hard and his lungs appeared congested on the chest X-ray. At first the congestion was thought to be caused by lung problems related to prematurity, but in a few days his heart was found to be enlarged and a soft murmur was heard. He was transferred to a heart center. After further examination and an EKG and echo-Doppler test, it was recognized that all the veins from his lungs were draining abnormally into the right side of his heart (figure 7.3) instead of into the left atrium. The heart surgeons thought it safer to let him grow a little bigger before putting him on the heart-lung machine. He was treated with doses of Lasix three times a day and transferred back to the nursery in his local community hospital for six weeks. Although his lungs remained congested, he was able to grow while on medication and receiving intensive newborn care. He had heart surgery when he was 3 months old; all the veins from his lungs were redirected into his left atrium. He went home two weeks later and was able to discontinue medications a month after surgery, since his lungs were no longer congested.

The heart may enlarge either because of a heart defect or because of disease of the heart muscle. When the heart is dilated and beating ineffectively, fluid may accumulate in the lungs and in the body tissues. Furosemide (Lasix), one of a class of drugs called *diuretics*, is often used for such children, who are in heart failure. Diuretics increase the excretion of fluid through the kidneys, thus relieving congestion in the lungs and in the body as a whole. Because furosemide also causes the kidneys to excrete more potassium and calcium than usual, the dose must be watched and adjusted, particularly in small babies or in children whose kidneys are not properly developed. Parents of a child who is receiving diuretics are often advised to give the child a supplement of potassium chloride, or to add to the child's diet foods that are good sources of potassium (for example, bananas, tomatoes, and raisins).

Digitalis, which is found in the leaf of the foxglove plant (figure 11.1), has been used in the treatment of heart failure ever since its discovery by William Withering in the eighteenth century. It acts by slowing the heart rate and by increasing the force of contraction of the heart muscle. Digoxin, a frequently used preparation of digitalis, can be given to infants as a pleasant-tasting preparation administered with a fluid dropper (marked to indicate the exact dose). Digoxin is an extremely valuable drug, but it must be treated with great care; even a small overdose can be dangerous. And, like any other medicine, it must be kept out of reach of toddlers, who might like the look of the pale green fluid and try it in error. Although digoxin in proper dosage occasionally causes mild stomach upsets, it is safe when given correctly.

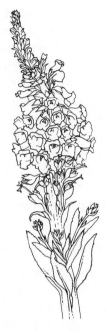

11.1.
The Foxglove Plant.
This plant is a source of the
cardiac medication digitalis.

In a few infants and children who experience severe or prolonged heart failure, another class of drugs may be used. After-load-reducing agents, as they are called, lower the resistance to the flow of blood into the arteries and small capillary vessels of the body. Captopril, the most frequently used drug in this group, is also sometimes prescribed when medication is required to lower a child's blood pressure.

Medications for the Treatment and Control of Arrhythmias

In a healthy child the heart rate varies with age and with the level of activity, but the rhythm is regular. When the regular rhythm of the heart is lost, an *arrhythmia* is said to be present. Arrhythmias include fast heart rate with abnormal rhythm (tachycardia); slow heart rate with abnormal rhythm (bradycardia); and other abnormal rhythms, such as long QT syndrome and extrasystoles. For some of these conditions medications are indicated, but about 90 percent of arrhythmias are extrasystoles and do not need medications at all.

Tachycardia

About 50 percent of all children who have one episode of tachycardia do not have another, but when the rhythm of the heart is persistently fast and irregular, there is a risk of heart failure, particularly in infants. Digoxin is often used to control attacks of tachycardia, but some children may need more than one medication, for example, quinidine, propranolol, or verapamil. Adenosine is another valuable medication now often used for babies. Although it rarely is, when the arrhythmia appears to be brought on by exercise, participation in strenuous sports or athletic competition may be barred. In severe arrhythmias, surgery or catheter treatment is sometimes advised when medications have not alleviated the condition.

In some babies there is no further trouble after the one attack, but in others repeated attacks of tachycardia do occur, and in such cases the infants will require continuing medication. Sometimes several different drugs will be tried.

Supraventricular tachycardia with heart failure

Robby P. was a healthy 3-month-old. His mother was at work one day when the baby-sitter noticed he seemed fussy and irritable and was not feeding well. He began to sweat as the day went on, although he did not feel hot or feverish. At home with his mother that night he was irritable, drank very little of his bottle, and was not his usual playful self. In the morning he was no better; his mother also noticed that his diaper was dry. She took him to the pediatrician, who counted a heart rate of 240 and said Robby had an enlarged liver and was in heart failure.

Robby was admitted to the hospital. An intravenous drip was started and ice was applied to his face; after the second application of ice his heart rate slowed to 120. He recovered quickly and was sent home the next day on digitalis. His mother was told that he had an abnormal bypass tract in his heart, or Wolff-Parkinson-White syndrome (arrhythmias and Wolff-Parkinson-White syndrome are described in chapter 8). She observed on a heart diagram what this term meant—he was liable to attacks of rapid heartbeat. Robby might have further attacks, or the abnormal conducting tract in his heart might disappear or quiet down on its own.

Robby was fortunate. He was able to stop medications by 1 year of age. He had only one further mild attack, around his fourth birthday, and was treated then as an outpatient. He is now 7 years old and extremely healthy, and he takes part in sports and school activities just like others of his age.

Robby illustrates an important and not uncommon problem: severe tachycardia with heart failure caused by Wolff-Parkinson-White syndrome. Robby may experience more frequent attacks as he enters his teens. He and his parents can then help his doctors decide on the best course of treatment. Teenagers may opt for surgery rather than continued medication, in which case electrophysiologic studies of the heart will be needed before a decision on surgery is made. Sometimes the abnormal focus that is causing the tachycardia can be treated in the catheterization laboratory and surgery will not be necessary.

In the two most frequent types of tachycardia in children, ectopic atrial tachycardia and reentry tachycardia, the normal sensitive controls no longer work, and the heartbeat is persistently fast. The heart muscle has great energy reserves but the heart will not tolerate these forms of extreme tachycardia indefinitely, over many hours or days, and heart failure may develop. Only one in twenty to thirty of all children who have atrial tachycardia ever need electrophysiologic studies, and only one in ten of these need surgery. But now that the types of tachycardia are better understood than in the past, almost all children can get relief from these troublesome attacks.

Ventricular tachycardia with long QT syndrome

Martha B., an active 7-year-old, was being chased across the playground one day by a classmate when a large teenager suddenly blocked her way. Martha collapsed on the ground. A teacher arrived and found that Martha's pulse felt weak and rapid, very difficult to count; a few moments later the pulse became normal. Martha was uncertain where she was or what had happened. At the local hospital later that evening she seemed normal, and no arrhythmia was found.

On evaluation the next day at a pediatric cardiology clinic, the EKG showed a long QT interval. Martha's parents were told that this abnormality meant she could have further attacks of passing out, and that she should start on beta-blocker medications if further tests confirmed the diagnosis. She was admitted for a stress EKG and some blood tests, and she began taking medication. She had no more attacks for five years. She is checked at six-month intervals to be sure that the dose of medication remains adequate as she grows.

Both of Martha's parents had the same syndrome in a mild form, but neither needed treatment. However, one aunt and one uncle had died suddenly in their teens while exercising, and a cousin was in the process of being treated for possible seizures. The cousin's EKG was also found to be abnormal; the cousin also began taking beta-blockers and her seizures stopped. She no longer takes antiseizure medication.

The combination of exercise and stress, as in Martha's case, may precipitate a serious ventricular arrhythmia, which can, if untreated, lead to sudden death. Most such children respond well to beta-blockers. Medication must be continued for life. A major international study of families affected by this condition is under way.

Most ventricular tachycardias in children arise from an abnormal focus in the muscle wall of the right or left ventricle. They are more dangerous than atrial tachycardias, because they may lead to ventricular fibrillation, a weak, disordered rhythm of the heart that does not allow the heart to beat properly and is quickly fatal. Ventricular tachycardias are rare in children with healthy hearts, but they do occur and may be troublesome. Careful evaluation in a heart center that specializes in childhood arrhythmias is essential. If a child's exercising brings on attacks of ventricular tachycardia, all competitive sports should be forbidden.

The long QT syndrome, which was observed in Martha, is an unusual condition that tends to run in families (see chapter 8). The child usually shows no sign of illness; a sudden fainting episode during exercise or when the child is acutely stressed or excited may be the first clue that something is wrong. The ventricular tachycardia in the long QT syndrome can be life-threatening. Because the QT interval fails to get shorter during exercise, as it does in the normal heart, a new impulse can travel down to the ventricle before the end of the T wave, during the "vulnerable period," and set off a run of rapid ventricular beats in quick succession. The underlying problem, the long QT interval itself, is thought to be caused by an abnormality in the nervous control of the heart, specifically the fibers from the left side of the sympathetic nervous system. For the occasional child or adult who continues to have tachycardia even while on medication, surgery to divide the abnormal nerve fibers may be advised.

Ventricular extrasystoles

Extra heartbeats (extrasystoles) are premature contractions that appear before the next regular beat is due. Are they a problem or not?

Sometimes these extra beats appear in the atrium, sometimes in the ventricle.

> *Mary has always been fine. They found these extrasystoles during a school physical. She had an EKG, an echo test, an exercise EKG, and a Holter test. All those tests! After all that time and expense they said Mary was fine. We knew that already. Why did they put her through all that?*

Premature beats in an otherwise healthy heart—beats not provoked by exercise—usually can be safely ignored. They are benign extrasystoles and do not need treatment.

Extensive tests such as the echo-Doppler are not needed for every child who has extrasystoles. Such tests are done when the extra beats are unusual in pattern and more frequent than in most children. The cardiologist will want to make sure that the heart muscle is working normally, since extra beats put more of a strain on damaged muscle than on a healthy heart. Exercise EKG and Holter tests can demonstrate that extra beats disappear with exercise. This is a good sign; if extrasystoles increase with exercise there may be an irritable unstable focus in the heart that requires medication.

> *Why is it that Don's uncle is on medication for his extrasystoles, but Don has just been told to drink less caffeine and forget about them?*

It turns out that Don's uncle has a lot of scarring or fibrosis of the heart muscle from a previous heart attack. Such extensive scarring makes the heart more liable to persistent extrasystoles or ventricular tachycardia, which can be very dangerous, so the uncle does need medication. Medication for ventricular extrasystoles is seldom recommended in children. Don is young and has a healthy heart, so he needs no treatment at all.

Tachycardia with mitral valve prolapse syndrome

Mitral valve prolapse syndrome is a term used to describe a small subgroup of youngsters with MVP (see chapter 9) who show an abnormal EKG response to exercise and experience frequent runs of tachycardia. Some of these children also show sudden changes in heart rate after only minimal exercise; others have a drop in blood pressure if they stand up suddenly (postural hypotension). Acute episodes of anxiety, or even panic attacks, may occur. Such children may need exercise testing and other studies to help decide whether treatment is necessary. Treatment with propranolol or a calcium channel blocker may relieve the symptoms of rapid heart rate. In rare cases, medications or biofeedback training may prove necessary for anxiety attacks. Graduated exercise training may be extremely useful in retraining the autonomic nervous system to respond more appropriately to sudden changes in position or movement.

A great deal of study is now under way to see whether such young people have some disturbance of the autonomic nervous system in either the sympathetic or the parasympathetic subsystem; these systems normally control heart rate, sweating, and a number of other "fright or flight" reactions.

There is a controversy about this pattern of symptoms. Some people in the field believe there is an entity, MVP syndrome, with symptoms directly associated with MVP; others believe that a few children or adults who have chest pain, rapid heart rate, and other symptoms happen to also have MVP. We do not take sides in this controversy but believe continued study is needed.

Patent ductus in the newborn

Medications to manipulate the ductus arteriosus have made surgery in early infancy far more successful than it was in earlier years. In certain heart defects—such as transposition and other conditions that cause cyanosis, and in severe left-heart flow defects—the baby does much better if the ductus, an artery joining the aorta and the pulmonary artery, can be kept open for a few hours or days after birth, while tests can be done and heart surgery arranged. Prostaglandin E1, which has been used for this purpose since the early 1980s, keeps the ductus open and has been crucial in the modern treatment of newborn infants who have critical heart disease.

For a premature baby in the first week or two of life, the drug indomethacin may make the ductus close, and surgery will often not be necessary.

Balloon Valvuloplasty

Pulmonary valve stenosis

Angelique P. was the child of migrant workers. She was born in Florida, weighing five pounds, four ounces; a heart murmur was noted immediately. She left the hospital at 48 hours old and had no regular medical follow-up. At eight months Angelique moved with her family to West Virginia. Because she seemed well but was growing slowly, a public health nurse arranged for her to be seen in the cardiac clinic in Martinsburg. There the cardiologist recognized that Angelique was in early heart failure and arranged an immediate visit for cardiac catheterization by Dr. Jean Kan in Baltimore.

Angelique had severe stenosis of the pulmonary valve. Her right ventricle was pumping at more than three times the normal pressure in order to get blood into her lungs. The myocardium of her right ventricle had thickened as much as it could and was beginning to fail. After balloon valvuloplasty the pressure in her right ventricle fell but was still higher than it should be. She was kept on propranolol for six months to help her overworked heart muscle relax. A year later she was growing and happy; she had a catheter test and the pressures in her heart were found to be normal.

Angelique's family said they had not realized how quiet she had been and how little she had played and smiled when her heart was overworked; only now did they recognize the difference. She had been a good quiet baby, with no energy to spare for play; now, after her valve was dilated by balloon valvuloplasty, she was a normal, active child.

Angelique's story is unusual. In nearly every child with pulmonary stenosis, a heart murmur is heard during infancy or early childhood, and after the child visits the cardiologist and undergoes echo-Doppler and electrocardiographic studies, the physicians can make an accurate assessment of the severity of the pulmonary valve narrowing (figure 11.2). Pulmonary valvuloplasty is discussed with the family as a treatment option for the future, to be done if the narrowing becomes worse as the child grows. It is very rare, however, for the stenosis to be as extreme as it was in Angelique.

Sometimes heart failure from pulmonary valve stenosis can be insidious, as it was in Angelique, and hard to spot. Babies with failure of the right side of the heart are not restless and irritable as are babies who have too much blood flow to their lungs. It was a wonderful series of events that led Angelique to receive what was then a very new procedure, just in time to save her. Now, in the 1990s, most valvuloplasties are performed long before there is any sign of heart failure, and no

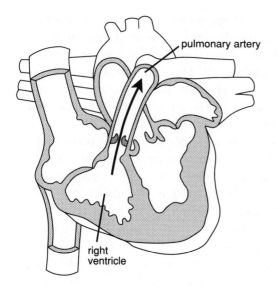

11.2. Pulmonary Stenosis. The pulmonary valve (*dark shading*) is thickened and narrowed, resulting in obstruction of blood flow (*arrow*) from the right ventricle into the pulmonary artery.

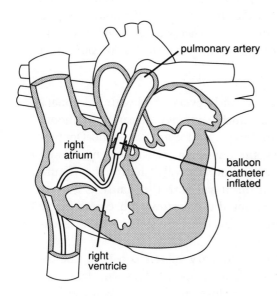

11.3. Pulmonary Balloon Valvuloplasty. Balloon valvuloplasty involves passing a catheter from the leg vein into the pulmonary artery. The pressures in the heart and the size of the pulmonary artery are measured, and angiogram pictures are taken. Then a balloon catheter is passed across the thickened valve, inflated, and rapidly withdrawn. The pressure from the balloon makes the valve open up; the pressure in the right ventricle falls almost to normal, since the obstruction has now been relieved.

medications are needed afterward. It is also unusual now for a child to need a follow-up catheterization, since the pressures in the heart can be calculated readily from the echo-Doppler test.

There is no need for any restrictions on the child's activity after valvuloplasty. Most cardiologists do recommend BE prophylaxis for such children, but the chance of their developing endocarditis is remote. Most children do, however, need to have a cardiac checkup every three to five years after a successful valvuloplasty has been done.

Fortunately, treatment of pulmonary valve stenosis is both excellent and safe. Soon after heart surgery became possible the valve could be treated surgically, and many adults who were operated on twenty or more years ago are now leading normal, healthy lives, often in strenuous professions. (One such person, a nurse, was a coauthor of a textbook that is widely used to teach medical students how to perform physical examinations on their patients.) The Natural History Study II found that patients with pulmonary stenosis did extremely well; twenty-five years after being diagnosed, about half of such patients in that study had had surgery and half had not needed an operation at all. Both groups were healthy and their life expectancy was almost exactly the same as that of their contemporaries who were born with normal hearts.

This good news became even better in 1982, when Dr. Jean Kan and her colleagues introduced the nonsurgical method of balloon pulmonary valvuloplasty to dilate the narrowed valve. In this procedure (which was used for Angelique), a special cardiac catheter is passed into the heart; the catheter has a balloon around it, and once the catheter is in the right place this balloon is carefully inflated. Pressure from the balloon opens up the valve to a nearly normal-sized opening (figure 11.3). The catheter is then removed; more pressure measurements are taken inside the heart and another angiogram picture is taken of the valve. The child is observed for a few hours in the same-day care center and can go home in the evening, having needed no anesthetic or hospitalization. Teenagers think much the best feature of the procedure is that there is no scar on the chest!

Treatment by balloon catheter has now replaced surgery for pulmonary stenosis. A recent follow-up study showed that stenosis successfully treated in this way does not recur. Surgery is needed only very occasionally, although it is sometimes necessary if more than one defect is present in the heart or if the valve is badly formed and does not respond to dilation by balloon.

Aortic valve stenosis

Daniel B. was born a healthy, full-term baby, but while he was in the newborn nursery doctors heard a heart murmur. During a cardiac evaluation and echo test at the local heart center, where Daniel's parents took him on the way home, he was found to have stenosis, a narrowing of his aortic valve. His parents were told that Daniel would grow and develop normally but that when he was older the narrowing of his valve might need treatment. He was as healthy and active as his kindergarten playmates, but an echo-Doppler test showed that the pressure in his left ventricle was too high (160 mm Hg); the pressure in his aorta was normal (100 mm Hg). The cardiologist said that this would be a good time to open up the valve with a catheter, so that the pressure in the left ventricle would not rise any further as Daniel continued to grow. Daniel went to the same-day care center and from there to the catheterization lab, where the pressures in his heart were checked and the exact size of the valve opening was measured on the angiogram. The aortic valve was then dilated with a balloon catheter; after this was done, the pressure in his left ventricle was down to 110 mm Hg and the aortic pressure remained normal at 100 mm Hg. He was admitted to the intensive care unit overnight, so that he could be carefully watched. No problems developed, and he went home the next day.

Daniel will continue to be seen by the cardiologist every year. His family knows that he may need another dilation, or perhaps even surgery for his valve, when he reaches his teens.

Although the role of balloon valvuloplasty is not yet as clear in the treatment of aortic valve stenosis as it is in the treatment of pulmonary valve stenosis, it is promising. With each month that passes, more infants and children with aortic valve stenosis are being treated successfully in the cardiac catheterization laboratory.

Aortic valvuloplasty is technically more difficult than pulmonary valvuloplasty, because the catheter must be passed into the heart through the artery in the leg, rather than through the vein. If the artery is small, as it is in an infant, the size of the balloon catheter may prove to be a problem. Catheter design is being steadily improved, however, and some infants and young children have already benefitted greatly from this method of treatment.

Medications are used for heart problems less often in children than in adults. This is so because most childhood heart problems concern the structure of the heart rather than the function of the heart muscle, and therefore surgery is more often the appropriate treatment. However, medical treatment can be of great value for certain problems. The use of medications for heart failure and arrhythmias was described earlier in this chapter. A single dose of gamma globulin given early in Kawasaki syndrome is extremely effective in preventing later aneurysms of the coronary arteries, and aspirin helps shorten the course of the fever and prevent clots from forming in the coronary vessels. Aspirin relieves the joint pain and fever in rheumatic fever and shortens the period of time during which the heart valves are inflamed. Steroids may be used instead of aspirin if the heart is severely inflamed, although there is still some uncertainty about whether steroids are more effective than aspirin in preventing long-term damage to the heart valves. Penicillin is prescribed to prevent future streptococcal infections and recurrence of rheumatic fever.

Almost all children who have heart surgery receive medications for a few days afterward. While they are in the intensive care unit they are often treated with diuretics and sometimes with drugs such as dopamine, which increases the rate and pressure of blood flow through the kidneys. After particularly complex operations, when the heart muscle may take longer than usual to recover its normal function, several medications may be used. After most surgery, by the time the child goes home, there will be no need for medications. At most, diuretics will be prescribed. After a heart transplant, however, cyclosporine is prescribed to prevent the body's immune system from rejecting the new heart. Many children who have had heart transplants also receive steroids, and sometimes additional medications are prescribed.

Children with Marfan syndrome may also be treated with propranolol. In addition to slowing the heart rate, propranolol eases the forcefulness of the heartbeat and is used to prevent the rapid progression of dilatation of the aorta, which is a particular problem in Marfan syndrome. Propranolol is also particularly useful in treating children who have arrhythmias of the heart and MVP; not only does it act to reduce the number of attacks of rapid heart rate, but it may also relieve the accompanying sense of anxiety or even panic such attacks can cause.

As new medications are developed for arrhythmias and suppression of attacks becomes even more reliable, it is likely that most children with arrhythmias will no longer experience frequent or recurrent attacks. As for balloon and other catheter techniques, they will supplant surgery for a few additional conditions in future years. The primary goal of heart research, however, continues to be the prevention of problems. The ambitious goal of a healthy heart for all children is always before us.

Chapter 12

Problems That May Be Treated Surgically in Infancy or Childhood

Certain heart defects require surgery within a short time after birth. (Critical newborn care is discussed in chapter 10.) Other defects require surgery but usually not until later in infancy or childhood. Virtually all of this surgery is performed before the teenage years.

Repair of congenital heart defects is increasingly scheduled by most heart centers for the first year of life. The reasons for performing the surgery early in life include the good effects of early repair on the heart muscle; prevention of complications caused by blueness (cyanosis), heart failure, or high pressure in the lungs; and an opportunity for the child to experience normal growth and play as soon as possible. The repair of many defects, however, can be performed over a wide age range.

With few exceptions, therefore, a "correct age" for surgery cannot be generalized; the correct age for an individual child can be determined only after the child and the particular defect have been reviewed by the health team and the family. This chapter provides examples of some of the heart operations performed during childhood.

The Principal Types of Surgery

Surgery can be outside or inside the heart (see the Introduction for a history of the development of these operations). In closed-heart surgery, the heart is usually not opened. In open-heart surgery, the heart is opened and the heart-lung machine is used.

Many people are interested in exactly how many children have heart surgery in infancy and how many have surgery later, during childhood or even in the teenage years. The number varies with different institutions and at different times. In our experience, of all babies born with heart defects who will ultimately require surgery, about one in four have surgery in the newborn period and at least one in four during infancy. In other words, about half of all heart operations are performed on babies rather than older children. This is a big change from earlier years, when surgery in infancy was much more risky than it is today and therefore was often delayed.

It is now quite unusual for a child to have a first heart operation after age 10, although for complicated heart defects that require several procedures, later operations, such as valve replacement, may be performed in the teenage years or even in adulthood. Today at least three in four of all children with congenital heart defects who will require surgery and who do not have this surgery in infancy will have been operated on before they begin first grade.

Closed-heart surgery

Closed-heart surgery, surgery without the heart-lung machine, is usually performed on the vessels around the heart, not inside the heart. Common examples include repair of a patent ductus or coarctation of the aorta (the Blalock-Taussig operation and other shunt procedures for cyanotic infants and children are other examples of closed-heart surgery).

In these operations the chest is opened by a cut or incision parallel with the ribs while the child is under anesthesia. The surgeon does not enter the heart itself. Closed-heart operations seldom involve much loss of blood, and children who have such operations recover quickly and usually go home less than a week after surgery. Such operations can now be done very safely, even on critically ill infants.

Open-heart surgery

In open-heart surgery, which is more complex, the heart wall itself is opened, or the surgeon operates on the coronary arteries. Open-heart surgery is employed to repair atrial or septal ventricular defects, aortic valve stenosis, tetralogy of Fallot, and other defects that cannot be corrected without making an opening into the muscle of the heart wall.

Because circulation of blood to vital organs must be maintained while surgeons are operating, a heart-lung machine is used to provide cardiopulmonary bypass. In most such operations, with the child under anesthesia, the surgeon opens the chest through the breastbone or sternum. Catheters are placed in the right side of the heart to drain blood from the veins into the heart-lung machine. The heart-lung machine, in a pump-like action, passes the blood over special filters that contain oxygen, whereupon the blood, now suffused with oxygen, is returned to the body through a catheter in the aorta. Because the heart itself has been bypassed and is no longer supplying the body with oxygen, it now contains very little blood, and it is possible for the surgeon to cut a small opening in the heart wall and repair the defect in the heart.

During the time on the machine (usually between forty minutes and two hours), the child's body temperature is cooled so the brain and heart muscle will require less oxygen than usual. In small infants under 1 year of age, profound cooling (*deep hypothermia*) is often used to reduce the body's needs even further.

Once the heart defect or defects have been repaired, the body's temperature is gradually increased to normal; the incision in the heart wall is closed and all catheters are removed from the heart, although usually one or more tubes are left in the chest for a day or two so that any blood oozing from cut surfaces can drain freely out of the chest. Often a pacemaker wire is attached to the heart muscle for a few days, so that a pacemaker can be readily affixed if any heart rhythm problems occur after surgery.

With modern methods of anesthesia, most children are awake, opening their eyes and recognizing their parents soon after leaving the operating room for the intensive care unit. While they are still attached to monitors, they are gently restrained from moving too actively in bed, but this time of restriction is usually very brief, often only overnight. Fortunately, although children experience pain in the chest wall after the operation, the pain is far less intense than the pain adults experience after a similar operation.

Although parents may well be alarmed at their first sight of the child in intensive care, attached to tubes and monitors, all tubes and wires are usually gone within twenty-four to forty-eight hours, and the patient goes back to a familiar room and begins to eat and move about in an increasingly unrestricted way. Many children who have had heart surgery go home in a week or less.

Ninety to 95 percent of open-heart operations are successful. If many problems exist simultaneously in the heart or the rest of the body, however, recovery may be less likely or may be long delayed (see chapter 14).

Heart surgery is now performed frequently, but it requires a major team effort and a special type of skill. The surgeon will explain to the child's parents exactly what the particular operation involves and how likely it is to be successful. Parents may want to visit the intensive care unit ahead of time to meet the nurses and look at the equipment. Becoming familiar with the surroundings and the staff will help decrease the stress involved in this difficult and anxious time.

Elective Surgery and Second Opinions

When elective surgery is recommended to prevent future complications, for example, when a child has an atrial septal defect or patent ductus yet is free of symptoms, parents frequently seek a second opinion. They may request advice on the timing of surgery, the best place for it, and the possibility of other options. Second opinions can be very helpful, particularly if communication between the family and the first cardiologist is less than smooth. Such difficulties are often due to style rather than substance; for example, the cardiologist may be an active and decisive person who implies that waiting another six weeks to close an atrial defect in a healthy 4-year-old would be morally wrong. In another case, a cardiologist who is calm and rather cautious may make the parents more anxious. They *want* to be told, Yes, now is the hour; no waiting, let's go. Hearing the first opinion confirmed by a second cardiologist, but delivered in a style more in keeping with their own psychology, can be quite reassuring. Also, the parents' insurance company may require a second opinion.

Substantive differences of opinion on elective procedures are now rather unusual. However, when a heart defect is rare and treatment is difficult there may be no real consensus on the best approach. Consulting with a center with particular expertise in a difficult problem may help parents and their physician decide on the best course. Most cardiologists are in constant touch with such centers and are willing to assist with referral to the best source of a second opinion.

A second opinion may not require a trip to a distant center. Often the cardiologist can send the results of the examination and studies (the EKG, echo, and angiogram) for consideration by the distant center's cardiologists. In fact, such a consultation is often obtained even when not requested by the parents.

Talking to Your Child about Heart Tests and Heart Surgery

Parents know their own child best, and so they are in a better position than anyone else to explain to the child what is coming up. It is usually a good idea to be very open, to explain that something needs fixing, and that it will be necessary for the child to be in the hospital for a few days. The child should be reassured that one of the parents will room in and the other will visit frequently. Pictures of the playroom in the hospital often help, and the child can plan what toys to take. Some parents, despite their own anxiety, manage to convey a sense of adventure. This is a great help to the child. In general, young children have little fear of death, and so they are more worried about separation than about the other aspects of being in the hospital. If they know their parents are close by and will stay with them, they come through the stay with few sign of stress.

We do not know how much children understand about their bodies, but even quite a young child may have an idea of the heart and circulation, as is shown in the drawing by a little boy 3 years old on the next page. Even so, elaborate explanations may lead to the use of unfamiliar terms, some of which may alarm the child. For this reason, parents are advised to use clear and simple language when discussing what lies ahead. We have found that when an adult talks to a young child about a stay in the hospital, simplicity, confidence, and optimism are the keys to a happy experience.

If for some reason surgery needs to be done in the teen years, the situation is different. It is quite important that the health team and the family discuss any possible risks with the teenager in frank yet optimistic terms. Sometimes an older relative has recently been hospitalized and has had many complications or even died. It is best to talk about what happened, not in detail, but stressing how different heart surgery is in a sick, elderly person. Some teenagers are helped by talking with another teen who has had a similar heart problem. Such a meeting and discussion can be offered, but should never be insisted upon, as individuals differ in how much they wish to talk to someone who is not already a friend.

At all times, the parents are primary in helping the child before, during, and after the stress of surgery. But the health team can make a valuable contribution to the triangle of understanding by allowing the child to have as much autonomy as possible and by keeping the child's safety, dignity, and happiness ever in the forefront of all treatment.

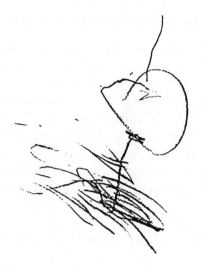

Courtesy David Bochner, age 2$\frac{1}{2}$

Closed-Heart Operations

Coarctation of the aorta

Ben W. had had a heart murmur since infancy, but he had grown well and was now an athletic 7-year-old. He was admitted to the hospital after being hit in the head with a baseball bat while he was watching his brother play in a Little League practice game. In intensive care Ben recovered consciousness quickly and was about to be sent to the regular ward when it was noted that his blood pressure readings were all higher than 120/90 mm Hg, well above normal for his age. This caused some anxiety, since a high blood pressure is sometimes a sign of damage to part of the brain. A pediatric resident felt the pulse in his leg and found it much weaker than the pulse in his arm.

A diagnosis of coarctation was confirmed by the cardiologist, and about a month later Ben returned to the hospital for repair of the coarctation. He did well after surgery, and went home six days later. The only complication was that his blood pressure remained higher than normal for several weeks after surgery, so he was kept on propranolol. After three months on medication his blood pressure came back to normal and he has not needed any more medication in the subsequent five years.

In coarctation of the aorta the problem lies in the area where the ductus arteriosus joins the pulmonary artery with the aorta (figure 4.5). Something has reduced the blood flow in the left side of the heart while the child was in the womb; the branch point of the aorta is narrowed where the ductus joins it. Before birth, this narrowing causes no difficulty; however, once the ductus closes after birth, either the left ventricle fails and there is an immediate emergency (see chapter 10) or the ductus closes off more slowly, as Ben's did, and heart failure does not develop in infancy.

Children like Ben may seem to be quite healthy. However, the blood pressure in Ben's arms, above the coarctation, was higher than the pressure in his legs, a difference in pulse and blood pressure noticed only after his accident at age seven led to an examination. A child with a coarctation may be so healthy that no problem is recognized until the teens.

Considerable research has been done on why the blood pressure is sometimes higher immediately after surgery than before. It is thought that when the abnormal flow of blood to the kidney arteries suddenly changes, hormones released from the kidneys elevate the blood pressure. Most physicians believe that there is a better chance of normal blood pressure in the long term, for the rest of the child's life, if surgery for coarctation is done in early childhood rather than in the teens or later. But surgery can be done successfully at any age. Almost half of all children with coarctation have a bicuspid aortic valve or other defect that may require treatment in later years (see chapter 4).

Repair of patent ductus

Walter E. was born in 1930. A heart murmur was heard when he was about 3 years old. He was healthy, but when his parents learned that heart operations were being done on children, they took him to Baltimore to see Dr. Helen Taussig. She diagnosed patent ductus (figure 4.3). Dr. Blalock repaired the ductus in 1943, when Walter was 13 years old. Except for a scar on the left side of his chest, he was then perfectly well thereafter. During the Second World War he was accepted for military service and sent overseas. In Paris he met and married a young French girl of 18 who had been born with tetralogy of Fallot, for whom a Blalock-Taussig shunt had been performed (she later had open-heart repair of her tetralogy and did very well). Their first child also had a patent ductus; surgery was performed in Baltimore when she was 5. Their second child had a normal heart.

Successful surgery for patent ductus has a long history, and as this true story illustrates, patients can lead completely normal lives afterward. It should be noted that if two people with heart defects marry and have children, the risk that a child will have a defect is probably close to 10 percent, so a decision to have children is not to be arrived at lightly. However, everything worked out well for the E. family.

Open-Heart Operations

Atrial septal defect

Annie K. was a thriving, happy baby. She was growing a little more slowly than her older sister had done, but at the age of 5 months she was sitting up and showed every sign of normal development. Her mother was surprised when the pediatrician said she heard a heart murmur and recommended that Annie be seen by a cardiologist. Both parents were concerned that it had taken so long for the murmur to be heard. The cardiologist diagnosed an atrial septal defect, which she showed to the parents on the echocardiogram videotape. She explained that the defect was unlikely to close on its own, but she recommended waiting until after Annie's first birthday for any surgery, to allow the defect a chance to repair itself.

At 15 months Annie returned to the heart center. The defect was still there, and a decision was made to do open repair. The operation was uneventful and Annie went home five days after surgery. She has grown well since then. She had two postoperative checkups, the first at one month, the second one year later. Her parents were asked to bring her back for her final check in five years' time. In the meantime she can live normally with no restrictions and no need for BE prophylaxis.

An ASD (figure 4.3) is a "moderate" type of heart problem. It can be found in a child like Annie, who appears perfectly healthy but who has been noted to have a heart murmur. Because such defects can lead to enlargement of the heart and abnormal heart rhythms in adult life, repair is usually recommended in early childhood.

Treatment of an ASD is usually by surgical closure. Although before the era of heart surgery many children with such defects did reach adulthood and some even lived to old age, a number developed complications of heart failure and high pressure in the lungs as they reached their thirties and forties. For this reason, and because surgery is both safe and curative, open-heart repair is usually done when the child is between 1 and 4 years of age. Most children can have the defect closed with stitches, and only occasionally is a patch needed inside the heart.

Although surgical closure of an ASD is safe, with a risk of any serious complication of less than 1 percent, it is still not easy for a family to adjust to the idea of surgery for a healthy, active infant like Annie. Some surgeons close the ASD by opening the right chest rather than by the usual breastbone incision. In girls, this scar will be covered up later as the breast tissue develops. Concern about the resulting scar, as well as the remarkable success of catheter techniques for treating other heart defects, such as pulmonary stenosis, has led cardiologists and families to consider using an alternative method of treatment. Several heart centers are now studying the use of a device to close atrial septal defects without surgery. The device, which looks like a clamshell, is introduced into the heart by a catheter. It is too early to say whether this device will replace surgery as the best method of treatment, however.

Will the atrial septal defect come open again?

No. Once the defect is well closed with stitches the endocardium grows and seals off even the little puncture holes made in the septum by the stitches. Very occasionally, less often than 1 time in 500, the repair is incomplete; if this occurs, it can be detected at the time of the first checkup after surgery and a decision can be made about further treatment.

I've never heard of an operation with no complications. Is everything as easy as you make it sound?

Complications can occur, but they are very unusual. When an ASD is repaired in a child over 2 years old or in an adult, fluid may collect around the lungs and heart between one and four weeks after surgery. This postcardiotomy syndrome is sometimes called *postpericardiotomy syndrome* (see chapter 14). Fortunately, such complications are very rare in children undergoing ASD repair. The most common problem is some postoperative arrhythmia; episodes of rapid heart rate (atrial tachycardia) sometimes begin several years after the operation. They are treated in the same way such episodes are treated in other children (see chapter 11).

About 95 percent of the children who have ASDs repaired have no complications. Serious complications, including death, occur in less than 1 percent of these children.

> *Why wasn't Annie's heart murmur heard until she was 5 months old?*

> *No one heard anything wrong in my little girl Janice until she saw a new pediatrician when she was 5 years old! Was her previous doctor deaf or something?*

An ASD murmur is not very loud, since there is no resistance to flow across the defect itself, and thus there is none of the turbulence that makes a loud heart murmur. Indeed, the murmur does not arise at the ASD itself, but rather is caused by the increased flow in the pulmonary artery. It is somewhat louder than an innocent pulmonary flow murmur. Some delay in diagnosis remains quite common, and Janice's defect can be repaired just as safely as was Annie's.

> *Will her children be normal? Will Annie be able to go through a pregnancy safely?*

A woman who had this repair as a child should have no problems with her heart during pregnancy and delivery. We usually recommend a heart checkup before the woman attempts to become pregnant, particularly if she has not had a checkup for five years or more. As for her children, the risk that a mother with a repaired ASD will have a child with this heart defect depends on whether other members of the immediate family also have defects. If the mother has no additional defects herself, and her own family and the father have normal hearts, any child of hers has between five and ten chances in one hundred of also having a heart problem. If a defect is present in her child, it is more likely to be an ASD than anything more serious (for more information on familial heart defects, see chapter 3).

Large ventricular septal defect

Carlos R. was a full-term baby, weighing seven pounds, two ounces at birth. He went home at 3 days old and seemed to be thriving. His parents were naturally alarmed when the pediatrician heard a heart murmur during Carlos's 4-week checkup. After some discussion everyone agreed to wait and see if the murmur improved. That evening he fed poorly and was fussy and irritable all night. His mother kept offering him her breast and he would start to feed eagerly, almost voraciously, for a few minutes, then turn his head and start fussing again. Was this colic, or did it have something to do with his heart? The family tried all the colic recommendations in their baby books.

Two weeks later Carlos had gained only two ounces since his last checkup. His pediatrician noted that he was breathing fast, that the murmur was louder rather than softer, and that Carlos was sweating even when lying still in his mother's arms. The cardiologist who saw him three days later found a large ventricular septal defect (VSD) (figure 4.3). He was started on Lasix twice daily by mouth. For a few days he fed better, but his weight gain continued to be very slow.

A cardiac catheterization test was done while the family stayed in the same-day care center; Carlos was not admitted to the hospital even overnight. The test confirmed that the VSD was large. The pressure in the lungs was three times higher than normal, and there was no sign that the defect was likely to get smaller soon.

At exactly 8 weeks of age, Carlos came in for heart surgery. His VSD was closed with a patch, and the operation went smoothly. He stayed in intensive care for two nights, then was discharged home four days later. He has now grown into a healthy, inquiring 5-year-old. His parents noticed that after he had been home from the hospital for a few days he "seemed like a different baby"; not only did he feed better, he had lost his irritability and stopped sweating, and his anxious look was gone. Now that he is in kindergarten, it is hard for his parents to believe how stormily his life started.

The delay in the onset of symptoms in Carlos seems strange at first; if this was a congenital defect, present at birth, why did he not seem sick immediately? We now know that this course of events is the usual one. We believe that in babies like Carlos, for a variable time after birth—often for several weeks—the small arteries in the lungs stay tight and constricted, just as they were before birth. The resistance in these small arteries is high and prevents much flow through the ventricular septal defect into the lungs. Gradually, as the small arteries in the lung mature and their walls thin, the resistance to flow drops; more and more blood goes through the defect into the right ventricle and the lungs become almost flooded with excessive fluid. At his catheter test, Carlos had almost four times as much blood going to his lungs as to his body. That is why he got so tired while feeding, and why he was growing so poorly.

Ventricular septal defect is the most common of all heart defects and accounts for about 25 percent of all heart defects found in infancy. More than 92 percent of infants with a VSD now reach their first birthday healthy. In about one child in five the defect closes itself, usually before the child is 2 years of age. In the majority it shrinks and causes no problem but a murmur. But if it is large, the child may breathe rapidly, especially when feeding; feed eagerly but quickly tire; sweat around the head; and grow more slowly than normal. Simple colds often turn into bronchitis or pneumonia.

Often, if a baby with this problem is not in severe heart failure, medical management at home will be attempted. If heart failure is present (as evidenced by an engorged liver, a pileup of fluid in the lungs, and a greatly increased heart rate and rate of breathing), or if rapid improvement does not occur with medical treatment, a cardiac catheterization test may be recommended.

The principle of treatment of a ventricular septal defect is to allow the defect a little time to shrink in size. But not too much time should elapse, because if high pressure in the lungs persists after a child's first birthday, the pressure never goes back completely to normal, even after successful surgery. So at the same time that medication is started to help move some of the fluid out of the congested lungs, arrangements are made to follow the infant closely.

The child's response to medication is sometimes quite helpful in deciding how urgent is the need to go on to heart surgery. Digoxin was used in the past in the medical management of babies with large VSDs; however, most physicians use it less often now because digoxin is primarily useful in stimulating the pumping action of the heart, and in most babies with large VSDs the heart muscle is already pumping effectively. The problem is that the harder the heart pumps, the more excess blood gets pumped through the VSD into the lungs with each beat, and the more congested the lungs become. Hence, a diuretic, such as Lasix, designed to increase the excretion of fluid through the kidneys, is now the primary medication.

Admission to the hospital for *medical* treatment is avoided if possible, because the risk of acquiring a viral infection is high, and such an infection can be very serious for these babies. However, if the baby is critically ill or needs oxygen, a few days in the hospital may make a big difference.

Almost all large VSDs can now be closed successfully even in very small babies, and when the defect is large and the infant is in trouble, surgery will be recommended, perhaps after only a few days of medical treatment.

Many times, if an echocardiogram and a catheter study suggest that the defect may get smaller over the next few weeks, waiting will be advised. In many babies some of the tissue around the tricuspid valve will grow over the defect and help make it smaller. (Because this tricuspid tissue forms a pouch or bulge over the defect, the term *aneurysm of the ventricular septum* is sometimes used; this is an unfortunate term, since *aneurysm* to many people means a bulge in the aorta or a brain artery, one liable to rupture. It is hard to associate the word aneurysm with a natural *healing* process!) It is a great triumph of modern surgery that if the defect remains large, surgical repair is so safe and so complete.

Other babies with large ventricular septal defects have a more troubling and difficult time. The doctors may place the child on medication for a long time in the hope of spontaneous improvement; for many weeks the baby may stay irritable and look thin and fretful. Other parents go through a bad time when a viral illness is passed around the family, for in the baby with a large VSD, a viral illness may turn into a major life-threatening illness requiring hospital care.

In a few cases, surgery may have been only partially successful, and the family must wait to see if another operation will be needed. The good odds for recovery are of little comfort when there is a sick baby in the home. Even more upsetting is the knowledge that in a baby who has several handicaps or a syndrome, the VSD is only part of the problem.

Once the VSD has been successfully closed, there are usually no more heart problems. Sometimes a soft heart murmur remains, caused by turbulent blood flow around the site of the repaired defect. In about one infant in ten a small residual VSD causes a murmur, but the defect is now too small to give any trouble. A recommendation about continuing need for BE prophylaxis can usually be made by the cardiologist at the one-year postoperative checkup. Abnormal heart rhythms are almost never a problem after repair of a VSD. In the early days of open repair, a slow heart rate was sometimes seen as a consequence of damage to the conducting system; this slow rate, or heart block, required pacemaker treatment. This is now a rare complication, occurring only in unusual types of VSD.

In children who have severe defects that produce signs of congestion and heart failure, medical treatment with digitalis and diuretics used to be the rule. Now, surgery in infancy is almost always the best course. This course has completely changed the outlook for infants with large ventricular septal defects. In past years such infants remained on medication for months or even years, growing poorly and often needing hospital admission several times a year, since any viral illness would make the congestion in the lungs much worse. Now a baby with a large defect of this kind is on medication for only a short time, long enough to see if the defect is going to get smaller on its own. If it does not, surgical repair is done, usually well before the child's first birthday. About 95 percent of these infants can be expected to live without medication after surgery.

Occasionally—in fewer than 1 baby in 200—a new murmur appears a few years later, a result of some tissue under the aortic valve. This *subaortic stenosis* may need treatment either by balloon dilation with a catheter or by another operation. However, the usual course is for a baby like Carlos to grow without further problems into a normal, healthy adult.

Multiple muscular/ventricular septal defects

Jerome M. was born with two strikes against him. He had several defects in the muscular part of his ventricular septum and his trachea (windpipe) was poorly formed and floppy, so that his breathing was noisy and difficult. He needed a tracheostomy to help his breathing, and he remained in heart failure. A band was placed around his pulmonary artery to reduce the torrential flow of blood into his lungs. After this was done, Jerome began to grow slowly. By the time he was 1 year old he had spent eight weeks in the intensive care unit and forty-four more weeks in the hospital, sometimes in a special chronic children's care hospital because he needed tracheostomy management. He was at home for only about three days before his first birthday.

Despite this bad start, Jerome was helped by a devoted family, who visited him frequently; by excellent nurses; and by his own sunny and engaging personality. Even at his worst, when every breath was loud and labored, he seemed to know that better times lay ahead. He was quite right. His VSDs gradually grew smaller, and he stopped needing any heart medications. When he was 4 his tracheostomy was removed, and he had another heart catheter test; it showed a tiny VSD that did not need surgery. The band on his pulmonary artery was removed uneventfully, and he is now active and playful, although he still wheezes a little when he has a cold because his trachea is still not strong.

Jerome's problem of multiple ventricular septal defects is unusual; it occurs in only about 1 or 2 in 100 babies who have VSDs. It was unfortunate for Jerome and his family that this difficult heart problem was complicated by the weakness of his trachea. Much of his need for prolonged care outside the home was caused by complications of his tracheal weakness and his tracheostomy, not by his heart. Every time anyone around him had a common cold, Jerome would develop a much worse infection, with bronchitis and wheezing.

Jerome's family was fortunate in that there was a chronic care hospital nearby that had developed special skill in managing tracheostomies, which in small babies can be difficult to manage. This hospital also had an excellent educational and social program for children. Someone outside his family visited Jerome every day and concentrated on helping him learn how to play with toys and interact with other children, and on helping him learn to talk in spite of his tracheostomy.

The precious years between 1 and 4 are vital: this is the time when the child learns how to interact with others and, even more important, learns speech sounds and what they mean. Because of all the special activities provided by the hospital, with the enthusiastic assistance of his family, Jerome was able to go to preschool and fit in well with other children. It would have been tragic if his heart had recovered but he had missed the opportunity for normal development and had not been able to fully enjoy his newly normal heart.

When there are several defects in the muscular part of the septum, it looks riddled with holes and is called a Swiss-cheese type of septal defect. These multiple muscular VSDs are hard to manage surgically, and some attempts are now being made to close the defects with the clamshell-like device introduced by catheter that we mentioned earlier in this chapter. Because this type of multiple defect is rare, any new treatment for it should be tested in a few major centers before it is attempted elsewhere. If a baby has this problem, parents need to confer with their health team about where their child can best be treated. In some babies staged operations may be recommended, as was done with Jerome.

Ventricular septal defect with aortic insufficiency

When Joshua P. was about 6 months old his parents learned that he had a ventricular septal defect and a patent ductus. When he was 3 years old a catheter test showed that neither the ventricular defect nor the ductus was large. After much discussion it was recommended that the ductus be closed, in the hope that the VSD would get smaller as Joshua grew. The ductus was closed successfully when Joshua was 3, but afterward his heart murmurs sounded louder than ever. He was followed in the heart center for several years, and it became clear that he had aortic valve insufficiency in addition to the VSD.

Valve replacement in children was still in its early stages at the time, so surgery was postponed until Joshua was 12. The VSD was patched closed and the aortic valve was replaced, since it was not possible to repair the leaking valve. Joshua is now 21 years old, a college graduate who regularly plays tennis with his father and his classmates. He takes anticoagulants (blood-thinning medications) every day to prevent the formation of clots on the valve, and his blood is checked every three weeks to make sure that the dose of anticoagulant is keeping the clotting ability of his blood in the correct range. In the eight years since his surgery, Joshua has had no complications.

Not everyone who has had a valve replacement and is on anticoagulants does as well as Joshua has done. It should be noted that if a little boy like Joshua were seen today in the heart center, the decision would be made to perform surgery when he was much younger.

A VSD with aortic insufficiency is an important variant of the commonest of all heart defects, a ventricular septal defect. In this variant, the aortic valve is involved in the VSD and gradually becomes leaky from constantly being pulled down into the defect with each heart beat. The problem does not occur with muscular VSDs, but only with those in the membranous septum or in unusual defects very high up in the septum. This type of defect can be very upsetting to the parents—they will have been told, quite correctly, that the VSD is small; then when the child is between 1 and 5 years old a new murmur, caused by the leaky valve, will be heard.

In the past it was hard to decide on the best time to operate on such a combination of defects. Usually the leaky valve got worse, and eventually a child who had started out perfectly healthy with a small VSD was facing heart surgery and replacement of the leaky valve with an artificial one. If surgery were not done when the child was young, the parents later would be faced with keeping a lively teenager on anticoagulants just at a time when the child hated to go near doctors and had an increased risk of injury and bleeding during participation in sports. The best course, therefore, is usually to operate early and repair the VSD as soon as the aortic valve leakage is detected. This course often prevents progressive damage to the valve. Whenever possible the valve should be repaired rather than replaced. This combination of defects, which occurs in fewer than 2 percent of children who are born with a VSD, needs particular care. For some reason, it is much more common in Asia than in the West.

Looping defect with large ventricular septal defect and pulmonary stenosis

Leonard M. was found to have a heart murmur soon after birth. He became a little blue when he cried vigorously, and he had many colds and ear infections in his first two years. He saw a cardiologist when he was about 1 year old, and an echo study and a catheterization test showed a large ventricular septal defect and pulmonary stenosis. The veins from his legs drained into an abnormal channel, bypassing his liver and entering the superior vena cava. The veins from his left lung drained normally into his left atrium, and those from the right lung drained into the right atrium. His liver was in the midline, not the usual right-sided position, and his stomach was on the right side of his abdomen instead of under his left diaphragm.

After the cardiologist described this long list of problems to Leonard's bewildered family and told them that Leonard probably had too many spleens, the family expected that he would be taken immediately to surgery. They were quite surprised to hear instead that everything was "balanced," that the pulmonary stenosis was protecting his lungs from damage by too much blood, and that it would be easier to repair his pulmonary veins when he and they had grown a little. Leonard had open-heart surgery when he was 4 years old and now, at age 10, is growing normally and doing well in school. He is not expected to have any future heart prob-

lems. He and his parents have been advised on how to keep him in good heart health during the years ahead.

Leonard, who also had a looping defect of the heart with hetero-doxy and polysplenia (see chapter 7), is a good example of a person who has an anatomic abnormality—in this case the route of veins from legs to heart—that is not of any importance and does not need treatment. Leonard had three other problems that did need treatment: the ventricular septal defect and the pulmonary stenosis needed repair to save the heart muscle from future damage from overwork, and the right pulmonary veins needed to be replaced into Leonard's left atrium to help protect his lungs from too much blood flow. In most babies with multiple defects, all of the defects can be repaired in a single operation when the child is between 1 and 6 years old. A different heart center might recommend that Leonard have surgery at a different time in his life, but such a variation is less important than the knowledge that careful analysis can often make clear exactly what needs treating and what does not.

Aortic valve stenosis

Ronnie L. was born with a heart murmur but was otherwise a healthy baby. He was diagnosed at 3 months of age as having aortic stenosis, and was followed up once a year. When he was 7 he had his second cardiac catheter test. The pressure in his left ventricle was now 190 mm Hg, the pressure in his aorta was 100 mm Hg, and his EKG showed signs of severe hypertrophy of the left ventricle.

Ronnie had successful surgery, an aortic valvotomy, and his left ventricular pressure fell to 120 mm Hg. However, the valve was badly formed and some aortic insufficiency (leaking of the valve) was found after surgery. He was well and active, but the cardiologist following him found that his heart was slowly enlarging and the leak of the valve grew worse each year. By the time Ronnie was 12 years old, it was recommended after a conference that the aortic valve be replaced. It was arranged that this would be done three months later. No further catheter test was needed, because the echo-Doppler test was clear.

While Ronnie was waiting for surgery he continued to go to school, but he seemed lethargic, he was not eating well, and he began to lose weight. He sometimes seemed a little warm and sweaty in the evening but had no other complaints. One evening he came home shivering and looking ill; he had a high fever. His pediatrician sent him back immediately to the heart center, where it was found that he had a bloodstream infection, bacterial endocarditis. The echo test showed clumps of clots and bacteria on his aortic valve.

After two weeks of intensive antibiotic treatment, Ronnie had surgery to replace his aortic valve. Ronnie's heart is now back to normal size and he is doing well again in school. He does need to take anticoagulants every day to prevent clots from forming on his artificial valve.

In aortic valve stenosis, the aortic valve is thick and domes upward with each heartbeat (figure 4.5), producing a murmur. The valve also makes a clicking sound as it opens. This combination of a click and a murmur is usually the only sign that the child has a heart problem.

In about one in twenty children with aortic stenosis, the valve is severely narrowed and badly formed and requires emergency surgery in the first days or weeks of life. In the past, however, because most children were completely free of symptoms, they might not be referred to a cardiologist until they were 5 years old and about to start school. Ronnie was 7 before surgery was necessary; by then his left ventricle showed signs of severe hypertrophy. Most children with aortic stenosis, however, appear healthy, and the presence of a heart defect is recognized when a physician hears a heart murmur, often with a click. The cardiologist will confirm these findings, and will use the echo-Doppler test and electrocardiogram to confirm the severity of the valve's narrowing and to determine whether or not treatment will be necessary.

The narrowed valve can be opened up surgically, as Ronnie's was in his first operation. Nowadays many children are having the valve opened up with a balloon catheter.

In the surgical procedure, which is called *aortic valvotomy*, the child is put on a heart-lung machine. The surgeon opens up the aortic valve carefully but not too widely. Because the shape of the valve is abnormal it cannot be opened up completely without making it leaky or "insufficient"; if a considerable amount of blood leaks back into the left ventricle with each heartbeat there will be a great strain on the heart muscle, and the ventricle will gradually enlarge and begin to fail. The goal of the surgery is to leave the valve with only a little obstruction and very little, if any, leak. After successful aortic valvotomy most children do extremely well for another ten to twenty years. Only occasionally does the valve need to be replaced in childhood. About one in three children do need to have the valve replaced later, usually in adulthood, because more narrowing has occurred with further growth or because the valve has developed more backward leaking or insufficiency. Ronnie's valve had to be replaced earlier, when he was 12.

Even in adulthood someone born with aortic valve stenosis needs a heart checkup every two or three years to make sure that the size of the ventricle and the status of the valve remain stable. One of the disturbing findings of the Natural History Study follow-up was that many patients who had been enrolled in the original study as children and had been brought back faithfully for many years by their parents had kept away from cardiologists once they became adults. Much of the responsibility for this avoidance of follow-up rests with physicians who have not made it sufficiently clear who needs to be followed. Certainly not all patients with murmurs do, but because aortic stenosis is a defect that may change and progress even in adulthood, cardiac checkups remain very important.

At a young age, probably in the early teens, the child with aortic stenosis needs to understand the nature of the problem. In the past the best course to be followed by a child or adult with aortic stenosis was unclear, and families often received conflicting advice on activity and wildly varying views on long-term outlook. Before heart surgery was available, a few patients with aortic stenosis died suddenly while exercising. The sudden death of a child with a murmur who looked well was not only an individual tragedy but a source of great medical stress and anxiety. Now that it is possible to see exactly how severe the obstruction is, physicians and families can collaborate in a well-defined treatment plan, free of anxiety about sudden catastrophe.

Why didn't Ronnie get an artificial valve at his first operation? Wouldn't he have been better off?

Sometimes, if the original valve is badly malformed, an artificial valve can save the life of a young child. But the artificial valve cannot grow as the child does, so Ronnie would have needed another operation anyway. Also, clots and infection are both more likely to occur on artificial than on natural valves. Keeping a young growing child on anticoagulants to prevent clots is a serious business and is to be avoided if possible, since it can lead to excessive bleeding in case of injury or surgery. Ronnie's natural valve served him well for many years. If a valvotomy (or now even valvuloplasty) can be done, it is always a better choice than valve replacement.

Could Ronnie's episode of endocarditis have been prevented?

The stenotic aortic valve is improved by surgery, but the risk of endocarditis remains. The aortic valve is less narrow than it was before surgery, but bacteria can still invade it more easily than they can a healthy and less delicate valve.

Clots on the aortic valve represent a serious complication, one that may lead to stroke if a clot breaks off and reaches an artery in the brain. However, it seems unlikely that Ronnie's endocarditis could have been prevented. It came on without any warning, and no surgery or intervention was done in the weeks before his symptoms appeared. The symptoms of bacterial endocarditis are often rather vague, as they were in Ronnie. Even after reviewing his history very carefully, the doctors could not explain why he had developed this serious complication. Endocarditis does sometimes occur like this, although probably two out of three attacks can be prevented by good dental care and conscientious BE prophylaxis (see chapter 14).

Subaortic stenosis and supravalvar aortic stenosis. In about one child in ten who has aortic stenosis the narrowing is *below* the valve. This *subaortic stenosis* is usually caused by a band of thick fibrous material like a form of scar tissue that lies about half a centimeter below the valve. The membrane is not a problem at birth, but it gradually gets thicker and forms a ring below the valve. It responds well to surgery and recently has been successfully treated with balloon dilation.

Most often, subaortic stenosis occurs by itself, without any other heart defect. Occasionally, however, a fibrous ring will be found to have developed in a child who has already had heart surgery for repair of a ventricular septal defect or in a child whose VSD is getting smaller on its own. In these cases, the murmur becomes louder than ever and the subaortic membrane can be seen on the echo study. In a rare tunnel form of subaortic stenosis, the obstruction is due to the combined presence of a subaortic membrane and a long tunnel-like area leading from the left ventricle to the aorta. Unlike the usual subaortic membrane, for which treatment is well defined and usually highly successful, this form of subaortic stenosis is quite difficult to treat and may require a combination of medications and more than one operation.

In *supravalvar aortic stenosis* there is a narrowing of the aorta one or two centimeters above the valve. This narrowing may occur in an otherwise healthy child, but it usually is part of a complicated problem known as Williams' syndrome (see chapter 15).

In spite of possible complications most children who have aortic stenosis become healthy and active adults.

Tetralogy of Fallot

George W. was the second child and first son of healthy parents. He weighed six pounds at birth and appeared normal. A heart murmur heard when he was discharged to go home was thought to be caused by a small ventricular septal defect, one likely to close on its own. George did well at home until one evening when his grandmother was baby-sitting; she noticed that he turned blue and began to breathe hard after taking only half his feeding. She tried to comfort him and finally he fell asleep after she held him over her shoulder, with his knees drawn up to his chest. When his parents returned he was sleeping peacefully in his crib. The next morning he was irritable and fed poorly. He was taken to his pediatrician, who again heard a murmur and detected some cyanosis of the lips and nail beds. A cardiac evaluation was arranged for the next day.

George was now 2 months old, a lively, alert infant who was normal except for mild cyanosis at rest. When he began to cry while being undressed, the cyanosis became more obvious. He weighed seven pounds, five ounces, and his growth chart showed that his rate of growth was slowing down. The murmur over his heart and the feel of a right ventricle tapping harder than normal all fitted with tetralogy.

During his echo test George slept peacefully and did not object to the cold jelly on his chest, or even to the sound made by the Doppler as it showed the fast turbulent flow across the area of pulmonary stenosis, the thickened muscle causing obstruction to the flow of blood into his lungs. A large VSD could be seen, with an overriding aorta (see figure 5.1). There was severe narrowing below the pulmonary valve, but the arteries to the lungs were nearly normal in size. The right ventricular muscle was thickened (hypertrophied). Thus all four features of tetralogy were present.

The cardiologist and the family looked together at the videotape of the echo test while George slept in the darkened room. He was now once again warmly dressed and held comfortably in his mother's arms.

George had a hemoglobin level of sixteen grams and a hematocrit of fifty grams, both higher than normal. Oximetry showed a nearly normal oxygen saturation at rest of 85 percent; when he cried the saturation dropped rapidly to 60 percent. Cardiac catheterization was done in the same-day care center, so George could go home after his tests and sleep in his own crib. No new defects were found during catheterization.

When he went home he did well for a few weeks, but then he had another severe blue spell in which he became very limp and breathed hard. He then became ashen in color and difficult to arouse. At the hospital he was given a dose of propranolol, and he quickly returned to normal. Surgery had already been discussed with the family, and it was decided that an early date would be arranged.

George was admitted for surgery for tetralogy at 4 months, weighing almost eight pounds. In surgery his temperature was cooled to 28°. On cardiopulmonary bypass the VSD was closed with a patch of Gortex felt, and the thickened muscle obstructing the flow of blood to the lungs was removed. At the end of the operation the pressures in all chambers of his heart were normal and the saturation of blood in his aorta was normal, at 95 percent. He returned to the pediatric intensive care unit, having been on cardiopulmonary bypass on the heart-lung machine for fifty minutes. He had been in the operating room for four hours. He did well after surgery, spending only two days in intensive care. He went home six days after surgery looking active, pink, and healthy.

Tetralogy of Fallot is the most common cause of cardiac cyanosis. It occurs in about three of every ten thousand infants born.

Although everything went well in George's only surgery, it was a stressful time for George's family. To them the two days their infant spent in intensive care seemed long and exhausting. When they got home in the evening the telephone rang constantly with inquiries, so they had little sleep. Once George was back on the infant floor they felt better; his mother was permitted to room-in, so she was able to watch his rapid recovery. His father went back to work but came to the hospital every evening while his wife spent some time at home with their daughter. The grandparents were helpful; not only did they baby-sit, but they provided loving support in many other ways. Another family who belonged to the local heart support group (Big Hearts for Little Hearts) acted as close friends and helpers during this difficult time.

As noted in chapter 5, the word *tetralogy* means that there are four defects in the heart. Only two of these are of major importance: *pulmonary stenosis*, a narrowing of the outflow area that connects the right ventricle to the pulmonary artery, and a large *ventricular septal defect* that causes blood to mix freely between the two ventricles (figure 5.1). There are also two minor or secondary defects. One is an *overriding aorta*: blood from both ventricles goes into the aorta, mixing blue venous blood from the right ventricle with normal, fully oxygenated blood from the left ventricle and leading to the baby's blueness or cyanosis. The other minor defect is a thickening of the right ventricular wall, called *right ventricular hypertrophy*; the large size of the ventricular septal defect leads to equal pressures in the right and left ventricles, and the wall of the right ventricle becomes thickened or hypertrophied as a result of this high pressure.

The more severe the stenosis, or obstruction, the less blood reaches the lungs with each heartbeat, and the worse the cyanosis. When the degree of stenosis is severe, cyanosis may be noted immediately after birth. In other infants cyanosis is not noticed at first, but a heart murmur may be heard, as it was with George. Sometimes this heart murmur is not very loud, and the infant may go home feeding well, to return later because of cyanosis. George had gone home and done well until the evening when his grandmother noticed that he had turned blue. George's grandmother was a good cardiac "detective"; she was the first person to notice George's cyanosis, perhaps because she had been around healthy babies and it was easier for her than for the young parents to recognize that George's skin had a slightly blue tinge.

The position of maximum comfort for George, the knee-chest position, is one often preferred by healthy babies, but it is particularly comforting to infants with tetralogy. In this position the return of blue (venous) blood from the lower part of the body is reduced; less blue blood then passes from the right ventricle into the aorta, and the cyanosis improves.

In addition to the other diagnostic tests, cardiac catheterization is still frequently recommended for such children, as it was for George, before heart surgery. A good picture of the small arteries in the lungs can be obtained, and sometimes additional defects not detected by echocardiography are identified. None were found when George was examined. It is likely that in the future, as echo-Doppler studies become increasingly sophisticated, fewer cardiac catheterizations will be performed.

The aim of treatment in tetralogy of Fallot is to restore the heart as nearly as possible to that of a normal child. It is a serious condition but successful repair in infancy is now nearly always possible. Repair involves open-heart surgery with closure of the ventricular septal defect and repair of the pulmonary stenosis (figure 12.1). The exact timing of heart surgery and what needs to be done varies from child to child. In George's case the surgery was performed at 4 months.

Open-heart repair in infancy, with no other earlier operations, is more and more often the recommended treatment. Repair is almost always successful. Each baby is unique, however, and the family, cardiologist, and surgeon will plan together for the best possible course.

About one in three of these children have another defect also, perhaps involving speech or learning, and this requires special treatment later.

Infants who have had surgery should have a cardiac checkup about one month after surgery and then a year later. If everything is well repaired a cardiac checkup every three to five years is often all that is needed. The echo-Doppler test is helpful in confirming that the ventricular septal defect is completely closed and the obstruction is gone. Except for BE prophylaxis, pediatric care and exercise can be normal.

Variants of tetralogy of Fallot are important, because they may affect the timing of repair and how much can be accomplished at one operation.

Tetralogy with pulmonary atresia. Tetralogy with pulmonary atresia is the most frequent and important variant of tetralogy. It occurred in one out of five infants with tetralogy born between 1981 and 1989 in the BWIS area. It is an important variant because it is much more difficult to treat than the more usual tetralogy with pulmonary stenosis, the kind George had. Also, babies with this variant are at higher risk of having additional problems outside the heart and are more often of low birth weight.

In pulmonary atresia (*atresia* means failure to develop) there is a complete blockage or obstruction of blood flow into the lungs, and usually severe cyanosis from birth. Sometimes the pulmonary valve is completely closed, sometimes the pulmonary artery is missing or replaced by a thin cord of fibrous tissue through which no blood can pass.

A.

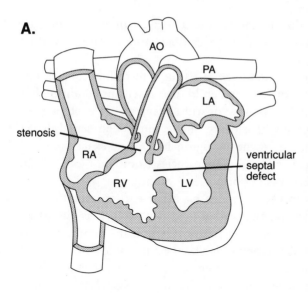

B.

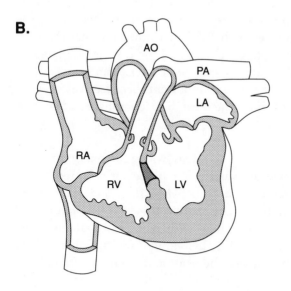

12.1. Open Repair of Tetralogy of Fallot. *A,* After the child is placed on the heart-lung machine the right ventricle (*RV*) is opened, and the ventricular septal defect and pulmonary stenosis and the pulmonary artery (*PA*) can be seen. *B,* The ventricular septal defect is closed with a patch of inert material (shown as shaded area), usually Gortex felt. The thickened muscle is removed from beneath the pulmonary valve and the valve is opened, relieving the pulmonary stenosis. If necessary a patch is placed over the front wall of the right ventricle to improve the flow of blood from the right ventricle to the lungs. The cut or incision in the right ventricle is then closed with stitches, and the child is weaned from the heart-lung machine.

Natalie L. was transferred to a cardiac center a few hours after birth because she was persistently blue, even when given oxygen. After many tests, including cardiac catheterization, she was found to have tetralogy with pulmonary atresia. She had some extra bronchial arteries supplying her lungs, so she did not need surgery immediately. Over the next four years she had two open-heart operations and a number of cardiac catheterizations, including one in which a special catheter was used to close off one of the large bronchial arteries.

Like many children with this severe type of tetralogy, Natalie had other difficulties: these included speech problems and a need for extra calcium supplements in infancy. Her parents and devoted family were well supported by her pediatrician throughout this anxious time.

Natalie is now happy and thriving in first grade and needs no medications. She is still receiving speech therapy.

Natalie's heart problem is less easy to describe than some of the others in this book, because it falls into a sort of middle range. That is, keeping in mind that the size and arrangement of the extra bronchial arteries varies widely between children (all the way from tiny to very large), we can say that if Natalie's bronchial arteries had been very small, she would have been intensely blue at birth, and her condition would have been discussed in the emergency newborn surgery section of this book. On the other hand, if her bronchial arteries had been larger than they were, she might have been very short of breath and she might have failed to grow, acting more like a baby with a left-to-right shunt.

It was fortunate that Natalie's bronchial arteries were large enough to let her grow awhile before surgery, and also that she was of normal birth weight. Not surprisingly, babies who are born prematurely and weigh less than five pounds at birth are more difficult to treat than larger babies. Natalie's greatest assets, though, were her family, her pediatrician, and the skill of those who performed the many interventions she needed, in the operating room and in the catheterization laboratory. Any baby born with tetralogy and pulmonary atresia has a challenging future ahead and needs the best possible help and a strong triangle of understanding.

How will George and Natalie differ from normal children as they grow?

Each will have a scar on the chest; if the family can accept this as a badge of courage, so will the child. There will be a soft heart murmur and minor changes on the EKG. Usually the tectrocardiogram shows some widening of the QRS complex, since the time taken for the electrical impulse to pass through the heart is longer than in an unoperated heart; however, this change is of no significance if the heart itself is well repaired and the heart rhythm normal.

The Timing and Prognosis of Surgery

The timing of surgery, as noted, is variable, depending on the severity of the heart problem and on the size and the condition of the baby. Heart surgery is now increasingly performed in the first year of life, thus avoiding strain on the heart muscle caused by the defect and avoiding complications from lack of oxygen or from prolonged high pressure in the lung arteries. Early surgery is particularly important for infants with atrioventricular canal defects or large ventricular septal defects who have high lung pressures.

Now that heart surgery is so much safer for infants than it was in the past, the focus of the health team and the family is increasingly on reducing the time the infant must spend in the hospital, and on making the child's stay there as easy and comfortable as possible.

Because most children after heart surgery can expect to live a long and healthy life, the family, the child's physician, and the cardiac health team will discuss the child's long-term outlook and the best ways of ensuring continuing heart health. Some children need closer and longer follow-up than others. Recommendations about exercise, schooling, and a heart-healthy diet can usually be decided upon within a few months after the child is home. Most children who have had open or closed operations can lead normal lives.

Chapter 13

Problems That Require Complex Treatment

The great advances of the past century have stimulated a need for better understanding of how and why heart defects arise. Surgeons have almost reached the limit of success with surgical repair of the most frequent defects, and it seems likely that the next big breakthrough will come in molecular biology rather than in surgery. Only when we understand why and how the left ventricle fails to grow in some infants can we hope to prevent and treat the worst heart problems. The overall picture of present treatment is immensely encouraging, in fact sensational, when you think of how far we have come. But a few conditions remain difficult to treat; some of these are rare, others very complex, and many involve abnormalities of the ventricles, which are the pumping chambers of the heart. Restoration of health in such situations may be hard to achieve, even after medications and surgery. Sometimes success will not be possible.

Major advances are still needed in the understanding and treatment of severe right- and left-heart flow defects. Although many infants can be helped through the treacherous period of adjusting to newborn life with only one good ventricle or pumping chamber, the long-term outlook for infants with such defects remains uncertain. The treatment and control of heart muscle disorders and cardiomyopathies also remain unsatisfactory.

In this chapter we provide examples of children whose heart problems required various kinds of medical interventions and procedures. Most of these children were born with underdeveloped (hypoplastic) right or left ventricles; the others had a variety of heart problems that did not respond to a single operation or medication and therefore required continuing and changing cardiac care.

In addition to hypoplastic ventricles, other congenital defects, including coronary artery anomalies and some forms of atrioventricular canal defect, may require a series of operations and treatments. The heart muscle disorders, dilated and hypertrophic cardiomyopathy, may need prolonged courses of several medications. Heart transplantation is the only treatment for some children with complex congenital defects or cardiomyopathies.

Complex Congenital Heart Defects

When an infant or child has a complex or rare heart problem that does not need immediate treatment, it is a good idea for the parents to check with the health team at a center with particular skill and experience in that problem. For example, there are three or four centers in the United States specializing in childhood heart rhythm disorders; a child's cardiologist will recommend that the child go to one of these if the usual treatments do not lead to resolution.

Hypoplastic right ventricle with tricuspid atresia

Warren A. was a husky baby who at birth appeared only slightly blue. But the oxygen level in his blood remained low, so he was transferred to a cardiac center when he was 3 days old. He was found to have tricuspid atresia, but he did not need surgery right away. He went home with his parents and did well for a few weeks.

By 2 months of age Warren was very blue. A cardiac catheter test showed that the opening between his right and left atrium was very small. Doctors enlarged the opening with a balloon catheter; then Warren had a Blalock-Taussig shunt operation (see figure 13.1) to increase blood flow into his lungs.

Warren grew well; it was difficult, looking at him, to remember that he had such a serious heart defect. He was checked every three months in the local county heart clinic. The original plan had been to wait until he was 3 or 4 years old to perform another operation, but six months before he was 2 the cardiologist became concerned that there might be too much blood flow to his lungs. Warren came back for another echo-Doppler and catheter test. The

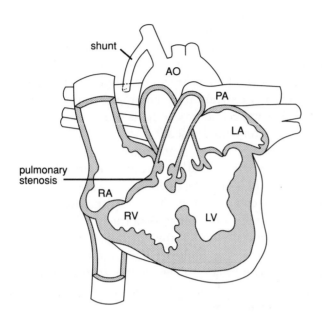

13.1.
Blalock-Taussig Shunt.
The artery to the arm, the subclavian artery, shown here coming from the aorta (*AO*), is divided and the end is joined to the side of the pulmonary artery (*PA*). This new shunt acts like a man-made ductus, allowing more blood to reach the lungs without going through the obstructed area between the right ventricle (*RV*) and the pulmonary artery. *Key RA* = right atrium; *LA* = left atrium; *LV* = left ventricle. (The heart defect shown here is tetralogy.

blood flow to his lungs was excessive and the pressure in his lungs was higher than it had been. Immediate surgery was recommended. In the Fontan operation the right atrium was stitched to the pulmonary artery, the previous shunt was closed off, and the opening between the two atria was closed. Warren had a difficult time after the operation; he accumulated fluid in first one lung then the other, and needed to be in intensive care for three weeks. When he finally went home he still had some fluid around his eyes and needed to be on medication and a special diet.

It was almost a year before Warren was back to his playful self. Now, eight years later, he is doing well.

Any baby with a hypoplastic right ventricle has a complex heart defect that may need several different procedures before health is restored. Some babies need surgery immediately after birth (see Amanda's story in chapter 10). Others, such as Warren, have a brief period of grace. The urgency of treatment depends on the flow of blood to the lungs. Warren's lung arteries were better developed and the blood flow to his lungs was better than is the case for many other infants who have hypoplastic right ventricle.

In children like Warren, who have tricuspid atresia, something has affected the flow of blood into the right atrium and ventricle early in fetal life and the tricuspid valve has failed to develop. The right ventricle is small because it receives little if any blood, and it can never grow enough to become part of the circulation. The aim of treatment is to provide adequate blood flow to the lungs with a shunt operation for a few years, and then to do a second open-heart operation to send blood directly from the veins and right atrium into the lungs, completely bypassing the right ventricle. This second procedure is called a *Fontan operation*, after the French surgeon who devised it.

The concept of the Fontan operation is an ingenious one. The idea is to bypass the useless right ventricle and to separate the circulation to the lungs from that to the body. When the operation is successful it results in a remarkable improvement in the child's health. However, it can succeed only if the pressure in the lungs is normal or lower than normal. Surgeons are still trying to modify this operation to make the postoperative course less stormy for children like Warren, who had high pressure in the lungs. The basic problem is the ventricle. When one of the two pumping chambers of the heart is defective, surgery can help but it cannot result in a true cure.

Many children who have had this operation do remarkably well. Warren and a number of other children who have had the Fontan procedure or a variant have taken exercise stress tests and been found to perform almost as well as normal children. The Mayo Clinic and Dr. Fontan's surgical group in Bordeaux, France, have shown conclusively that some children with a hypoplastic right ventricle can become healthy and active participants in life. Each individual success like Warren's represents a triumph over this severe and formerly always fatal heart defect.

Hypoplastic left ventricle with later cardiomyopathy of the right ventricle

Kenneth B. was born with a severe heart defect, hypoplastic left ventricle. He had an operation when he was several days old, after which his color became almost normal and he began to grow slowly. However, the cardiologists who saw him noticed every time they checked him that his right ventricle, his only "good" ventricle, was steadily enlarging. Even worse, the function of the ventricle was getting weaker.

At about 13 months Kenneth began to lose ground; he was feeding poorly and was not gaining weight, and he was tired and irritable all the time. After much discussion over the next two months, a heart transplant was performed when he was 15 months

*old. He has continued on several medications, including pred-
nisone and cyclosporine. During the first year after the operation
he came to the hospital every month for a heart biopsy. The family
stayed at the same-day care center each time, since their home
was some distance away.*

*Kenneth was in the hospital for several days on three occa-
sions between the ages of 18 months and 3 years because of
episodes of rejection of the new heart. At 5 years old, he was doing
well and required a biopsy only twice a year. He had not been hospitalized for almost two years. He was lively and very active.*

*Kenneth died suddenly at the age of 5 from thickening or ath-
erosclerosis of the coronary arteries, one of the problems that
sometimes occurs in children who have had transplants. His parents were grateful for the good years he had had, and they helped
produce a wonderful booklet for other families like their own, for
whose child a heart transplant is one method of treatment.*

Kenneth was born with a hypoplastic left ventricle and then developed severe heart muscle failure, a form of cardiomyopathy. Either
problem may lead doctors to consider a transplant. Kenneth had both
problems.

A heart transplant is one of the first operations considered for infants who have hypoplastic left ventricle, but there is at present no consensus that transplant is the treatment of choice. No one else can fully
enter into the agonizing decision that must be faced by the families of
such children. The fact that a transplant is considered does not necessarily mean that it can or should be done. Apart from questions of
donor supply and timing (the concern over whether there will be an
appropriate heart available when the transplant is needed), the follow-
up period involves a great deal of parental time and effort, and this
commitment will not be possible for every family. Kenneth's parents
feel that they made the right decision for their own set of circumstances.

Endocardial cushion defect requiring two operations

*Laura O. had grown rather slowly but had no other symptoms.
When she was 3 years old she was sent to a cardiologist to find out
whether her slow growth was related to a soft heart murmur that
had recently been noticed. Echo tests were not yet available at that
time, but the type of murmur and the unusual electrocardiogram*

made the cardiologist suspect Laura had an endocardial cushion defect. This suspicion was confirmed at cardiac catheterization; she did not have the most severe form of the defect, but instead had an abnormal leaking mitral valve in addition to a defect in the lower part of the atrial septum. The atrial septal defect was surgically closed and the mitral valve was repaired with some stitches.

After surgery, although Laura grew well and was very active, the heart murmur suggested that her mitral valve was still leaking quite badly. By the time she was 15 years old her heart had become very large; after further tests her mitral valve was replaced. She improved greatly, but of course needed to be on anticoagulants to prevent clots from forming on her artificial valve.

Laura was conscientious in coming for follow-up visits. She became pregnant when she was 20 years old and had a healthy little boy. Her use of anticoagulants needed to be carefully supervised during this time. Three years later she became pregnant again, and this time the baby, Lauretta, had both Down syndrome and an endocardial cushion defect. The heart defect was successfully repaired and Lauretta is doing well in a special education program.

Laura's story shows that endocardial cushion defects can still present problems. Laura had a partial atrioventricular canal defect, while Lauretta had the more severe complete form illustrated in figure 6.1. Almost all children with incomplete forms of the defect (sometimes called an ostium primum defect) now do well after only one operation, which is usually performed when the child is between 1 and 4 years of age. The newer methods of repairing the mitral valve are better now than those used in the past, but some valves defy the best surgical attempts.

Laura's story also illustrates the great need to follow families through to the next generation. A fetal echocardiogram and other tests are usually recommended for a pregnant woman who has a heart defect. The surgical treatment of endocardial cushion defects has advanced more rapidly than understanding of how they develop and what relationship they have to defects in other parts of the body. Prevention of such defects, particularly when they are associated with other severe problems such as Down syndrome, remains an important goal.

Successful repair of the more severe complete form of atrioventricular canal defect, the kind Lauretta had, remained a surgical challenge for many years, not only because the severity of the malformation made surgical correction technically difficult, but also because of the frequent complication of rapidly developing damage to the small lung arteries in response to high pressure in the pulmonary artery. For a number of years, surgery in infants was technically too difficult, yet by the time the child was big enough for safe surgery, the pressure in the lungs was high and would not drop even if the defect was repaired. The aim of treatment now is to close the defect and repair the valves in infancy (usually before the child is 6 months old), before the lung pressure gets too high for safe surgery. In most babies the diagnosis is made in the first month of life. If lung congestion and breathing difficulty develop, the child is treated with furosemide (Lasix) for a few weeks or months. Open heart repair is done using the heart-lung machine and cooling (hypothermia). The defects in both the atrial and the ventricular septum are closed; some surgeons use two separate patches, others "tailor" a single patch to close the large irregularly shaped hole in the center of the heart. Repairing the valves is the most difficult and delicate part of a very difficult operation.

In many centers this operation is done with a high success rate; despite the technical challenges, about nine times out of ten the infant's condition can be improved to a remarkable degree, and cardiac medications can be discontinued within a few weeks after the child's discharge from the hospital. A very few children may have problems after surgery. These include the development of abnormal heart rhythms and the appearance of narrowing below the aortic valve. *Heart block*, a slow heart rhythm requiring pacemaker treatment, was common when repair of atrioventricular canal defects first began, because of the disturbed route taken by the conducting system. Today this complication is unusual.

Some children develop a new murmur because of obstruction below the aortic valve—subaortic stenosis. The most frequent complication is a progressive worsening of the leak or insufficiency of the mitral valve after the original surgery; in about 1 in 100 of these children replacement of the mitral valve is necessary later, sometimes many years after the original repair, as happened in Laura. All in all, careful postoperative checks are even more essential for a child after surgery for an atrioventricular canal defect than for most other children.

However, the overwhelming majority of children with endocardial cushion defects, who have no additional defects outside the heart, grow well after surgery and can live actively and free of restrictions. BE prophylaxis is always needed, because the valve leaflets are never completely smooth even after repair.

Abnormal origin of the left coronary artery from the pulmonary artery

Betty J. was born in 1956. She was a healthy baby until she was 2 months old, when she began to have attacks of screaming and sweating during feeding. Her formula was changed several times but the attacks continued. Her mother brought Betty to the hospital because she was breathing fast and sounded wheezy. A chest X-ray showed an enlarged heart, so large that it was pressing on the lower part of the left lung, and causing Betty to wheeze. Betty was referred to a cardiologist, who did an EKG and a cardiac catheter test; they showed that the left coronary artery arose from the pulmonary artery, not from the aorta as it normally does.

At that time, no one had been able to operate successfully on the coronary arteries, even in adults. But some surgeons thought the small extra coronary branches would grow if the pericardium, the lining of the outside of the heart, was irritated or inflamed. Therefore, after a great deal of discussion, the surgeons opened Betty's chest and placed some phenol and talc on the pericardium to cause irritation. She convalesced slowly, had no more screaming attacks, and grew into a normal child and adult, although her heart remained large and her EKG still showed evidence of some dead heart muscle. She married at 28 and had a healthy baby.

Soon after her baby was born, however, Betty began to be bothered by abnormal heart rhythms—multiple runs of extrasystoles—which kept her awake, and she was admitted to the hospital for another heart catheter test. She had a second operation, this time with a heart-lung machine. The left coronary artery was replaced into the aorta. Although her EKG is still not normal, she now has a less abnormal heart rhythm. Now, eight years after this second operation—and thirty-six years after her serious heart defect was discovered—she is a healthy and active member of her family, her church, and her community.

In this book we have tried to tell the medical stories of babies who typify the usual course of a heart problem. Betty is completely atypical; her first operation had been done only a few times and no one could be certain how well she might have done with medical treatment. Those of us who saw her as a sick infant, were certain that without surgery she would die in a few days or weeks, as we had seen so many other similar babies do, but no one could predict this for sure. We chose to tell her story because she has remained a friend and a source of support, someone who encouraged us in writing this book when few others did so. Her story demonstrates that at different stages in life our roles can change; the former patient becomes the friend and gentle counselor. Betty and all of us also owe much to her devoted parents, who were not deterred by the problems of inner-city Baltimore life and gave her every chance they could.

An infant with this rare coronary artery defect seems quite healthy at birth and usually has no heart murmur or any symptom to direct attention toward the heart. During the early months of life, however, trouble begins. As the pressure in the lung arteries falls, blood starts to flow backwards—*down* the right coronary, in the normal way, but backward *up* the left coronary to the pulmonary artery (figure 7.5)—in what is often described as a "coronary steal"; that is, good oxygen-containing blood is being stolen from the heart muscle by the abnormal flow into the pulmonary artery. The first symptom is usually difficulty in feeding. Usually at an age of between 3 and 6 months (for Betty it was 2 months) the infant stops feeding eagerly and often cries and seems colicky after feeding only a few minutes.

The chest X-ray confirmed that Betty's heart was larger than normal. In cases like Betty's, the EKG may show a very specific set of changes, exactly like those seen in a middle-aged person having a severe heart attack. This "infarct pattern" on the EKG occurs because the heart muscle of the left ventricle is not getting enough oxygen and nutrients; the blood that should supply the muscle is going into the pulmonary artery, being "stolen." So even though the baby is only 2 or 3 months old, some of the muscle of the vital left ventricle is dead or dying. Betty's EKG showed evidence that some of her heart muscle had died.

In an infant born today with a heart defect like Betty's, an echo-Doppler will show three important findings: first, the enlargement of the right coronary artery, which has dilated to try to increase the flow of blood to the damaged heart; second, the extent of damage to the heart muscle; and third, the abnormal course of the blood flow, which can be tracked back up into the pulmonary artery (figure 7.5). Cardiac catheterization is sometimes needed if the echo-Doppler findings are not conclusive, or if some additional defect is suspected.

In children with abnormal origin of the left coronary artery it would seem very logical to operate immediately, replacing the left coronary artery into the aorta, thus preventing any further damage to the heart muscle. However, this course is not always recommended. The debate about management is based on the fact that the extent of damage to the heart muscle varies from child to child and the part of the muscle that is already dead will not recover, whereas damaged or dying muscle can be restored once the blood supply is normal. Some babies benefit from medical treatment, with delay (usually of a few weeks' or even months' duration) of the surgery that will rejoin the coronary artery to the aorta. The debate is based also on the fact that this defect is rare and varies greatly in severity; no one can be certain of the best course to take. Occasionally, in an infant who seems very sick and has serious damage to the heart muscle, a brief operation will be done to ligate, or tie off, the left coronary artery and abolish the "coronary steal." Some surgeons have found even the best results of operations to move the coronary artery so discouraging that they recommend heart transplantation if the area of dead muscle is extensive.

Cardiomyopathy

Tab H. had a healthy childhood and was a good football player. At 16 he felt he was not able to run as long or as hard as he had a year before, but he told nobody and remained on the high school team. One day he collapsed during a practice game and was brought to the hospital. His heart was found to be quite enlarged; echo testing showed that the heart muscle was not contracting or beating with the strength or force normal in a young boy.

Tab had a cardiac catheterization and a small sample of heart muscle was removed through the catheter in an endomyocardial biopsy. Microscopic study of the biopsy showed fibrous scarring (fibrosis) of the muscle (the myocardium) and, in addition, a remarkable thickening of the inner lining of the heart (the endocardium). Everything suggested that Tab had had an inflammation of the heart in infancy, followed by progressive scarring. Tab now had a large dilated heart, or dilated cardiomyopathy. Despite the use of many medications, Tab's heart function showed little improvement. About eighteen months after his first admission to the hospital he underwent a cardiac transplantation and has done well since then.

Tab's is a true and rather alarming story, illustrating that in a few rare cases, a teenager can appear well and yet have a serious heart disease. Tab most likely had had a "silent" viral infection of the heart before or shortly after birth, and this infection led to more and more scarring. Eventually most of his heart muscle was replaced by scar tissue (fibrosis).

If a child nowadays has viral myocarditis and there are signs that the heart muscle is being damaged, a heart biopsy may be done. (This was not done on Tab for two reasons: the viral illness we think he had did not give any sign that it was affecting his heart, and when Tab was a baby, heart biopsies were not yet being performed on young children.)

A heart biopsy may be done if there are any signs that the function of the myocardium is being damaged. In an effort to contain the invasion of the virus, the body is actually turning on itself, making antibodies that cause fibrous scarring of the myocardium. If the biopsy shows an acute change in the muscle cells, steroids and other drugs to suppress the immune response may be prescribed. Although it is not yet certain how often this vigorous treatment succeeds, so far it seems promising.

> *Why did Tab respond to a virus this way? Is anyone else in the family likely to get the same thing?*

Many investigators are looking for genetic markers that might show how Tab, for example, differed from others who were exposed to the same virus but were not harmed by it. There is some sign of minor differences in genetic typing between cardiomyopathy-prone families and others, but there is no clear answer yet on the risk of any one individual.

Viral myocarditis, which Tab apparently had contracted before or shortly after birth, is an inflammation of the heart muscle caused by a viral infection. The inflammation may heal completely, leaving no sign of damage, or it may result in mild scarring that will show up on an echo test or electrocardiogram, even though the child has grown into a healthy adult. Or, as happened to Tab, there may be permanent damage and progressive scarring. Tab is still doing well about six years after transplant.

Of the children who have viral myocarditis, some will recover completely and some will have mild long-term effects, but only a very few will develop cardiomyopathy. Because cardiomyopathy is so serious, much research is under way to see whether vigorous treatment of myocarditis will help the heart heal completely.

Heart Transplants and Heart-Lung Transplants

Children who undergo heart transplantation have had either cardiomyopathy or very complex congenital heart defects. When medical management of cardiomyopathy leads to no improvement, and when use of diverse medications does not successfully control heart failure, transplantation is a good, though never an easy, option.

Heart transplantation can dramatically improve a child's life, transforming a child who is chronically ill and weak to one capable of almost normal activity and growth. Because of the need for many postoperative medications, the constant risk of rejection, and the unknown long-term side effects, however, heart transplantation poses many difficulties for the child, the family, and the health team.

Transplantation almost always leads to chronic rejection of the new heart; this rejection is itself a form of cardiomyopathy. The problems accompanying rejection of the new heart tissue, which were once overwhelming, can now be much better controlled by adding cyclosporine to the drugs used postoperatively. About 200 heart transplants have been performed in children; the present survival rate one year after transplant is 85 percent and the expected five-year survival rate is 74 percent.

Heart-lung transplantation is considered only when the child's heart is badly diseased and the lungs are damaged by high blood pressure or by a chronic illness such as cystic fibrosis. However, the results of heart-lung transplantation in children to date have been less promising than those of heart transplantation alone.

Many institutions that have heart transplant programs for children have developed excellent family-oriented booklets describing how a child is followed up medically in their institution, how often the child needs to come back for tests, and the special points the family needs to know about infections or fever. The booklet used at Johns Hopkins was prepared by the transplant team with much help from families, and it contains some lovely photographs of children and parents at different times before and after surgery. Such booklets can be very helpful.

Chapter 14

Complications of Childhood Heart Problems

Most children with heart problems do well and do not develop complications of any kind. In a few children complications may arise in the heart itself, or from effects of the heart problem on other parts of the body, or as a result of treatment.

All medications and operations carry some risk, and the health team and family need to review these risks carefully together. However, complications after surgery are steadily decreasing every year, now that operations are done earlier and now that techniques for protecting the heart muscle and the brain have become more sophisticated.

When either medical or surgical treatment is required, the family needs to become well informed about possible complications and their symptoms.

Possible Medical Complications

Larry G. had been healthy in early infancy, but at 7 months old he became fussy while feeding, stopped being as playful as before, and looked a little puffy around the eyes. His physician found that his heart rate was 140 all the time; it did not vary with activity, as is normal. She also noticed some enlargement of the liver, and she suspected mild heart failure. The cardiologist agreed that Larry had supraventricular tachycardia caused by an ectopic focus in the atrium, and she prescribed digoxin and quinidine. Larry's heart rate slowed to about ninety, and he was much happier and

225

eating like his old self; however, about a week later he developed a rash and some blotching of the skin that looked like bruising. His parents had been warned that some children react this way to quinidine, and after they talked to the physician they stopped the quinidine. A few days later Larry began treatment with propranolol, in addition to digoxin. He has remained out of heart failure and free of other complications for two years.

Larry's story illustrates two different types of complications: first, the slow onset of heart failure, a complication of tachycardia before treatment, and a rash and bruising caused by the quinidine that had been used to treat the tachycardia. Sometimes several medicines for arrhythmias will have to be tried before one is found that controls the abnormal focus and yet does not produce unacceptable side effects.

All medications have some side effects. Nevertheless, complications of treatment for childhood heart disorders are quite rare, and almost all such complications can be detected early and successfully treated.

The health team and the pharmacy should carefully review the potential side effects of medications with the parents before medication is begun. For example, vomiting is a sign of toxic side effects from digoxin, but it can also be a sign of heart failure; therefore, the parents need to be told how to proceed if a baby who is taking digoxin vomits or refuses food. The plan should be written down, so that there will be no confusion about what to do if this happens.

An infant cannot describe his or her symptoms. An adult who has a low level of potassium in the blood from excessive diuretics will complain of fatigue and muscle weakness, but a sick baby with a similar problem can only cry a little harder or act a little more cranky. We have found that a change in the usual pattern of the child's behavior is the best sign for parents to look for. Often it takes several visits to the child's physician and some extra blood tests to determine whether a new medication is or is not the cause of new symptoms.

Any medication used to treat arrhythmia may have complications of its own, ranging from "beta-blocker blues," caused by propranolol and related drugs, to an occasional paradoxical *increase* in severity of arrhythmia, caused by certain new drugs such as flecainide. Because the most potent of the anti-arrhythmic drugs, amiodarone, may have many side effects on the lungs and on liver function—effects that, fortunately, seem to be rarer in children than in adults—this drug is recommended only if arrhythmia is severe and prolonged. Before starting any of this group of medications the family and health team should review together exactly what side effects may occur and how they should be handled.

Possible Surgical Complications

As surgical techniques in heart surgery have advanced, the number and severity of complications have declined dramatically. Possible complications of surgery are usually discussed with the family in detail at the time parental consent for surgery is obtained. The specific risk of the procedure and the type of potential complications vary from one operation to another, and they need to be understood by the parents.

Immediate postoperative problems, such as bleeding, acute failure of the heart or kidneys, or collapse of part of a lung, usually occur in the first two days following the operation if they occur at all. Other postoperative complications that may occur include arrhythmia, infection, postpericardiotomy syndrome, and neurologic disorders.

Arrhythmias

Arrhythmias (abnormal heart rhythms) are probably the most frequent complications of heart surgery. Arrhythmias may occur while the child is in intensive care or, more rarely, several years after successful heart surgery. The type of arrhythmia and its frequency depend on the nature of the underlying heart problem, the operation performed, and even on the historical period in which surgery was done. For example, a slow heart rhythm, or heart block, was a major complication in the early days of repair of ventricular septal or endocardial cushion defects; this condition was due to damage and scarring of the specialized muscle fibers of the conducting system that carry electrical messages regarding heart rhythm between the atrium and ventricle. Some children needed permanent pacemakers after surgery. Nowadays heart block, if it occurs at all, is almost always due to simple bruising or swelling around the conducting fibers, and it disappears after a few days. Pacemaker wires are left in the heart muscle at the end of the operation, so that any slow rhythm can be treated easily; the wires are removed before discharge from the hospital. Other arrhythmias that occur immediately postoperatively usually can be treated with medication and are resolved by the time of the child's discharge from the hospital.

If the child complains of a thumping or pounding in the chest long after surgery, arrhythmias can be suspected. Or they may be recognized by the school nurse or the child's physician. Although not all arrhythmias require treatment, it is usually prudent to have them checked out.

Children who have had an atrial switch (Mustard or Senning) operation for transposition or a Fontan procedure (see chapter 13) for a complex heart defect are very likely to have atrial arrhythmias, and they may have slowing of the heart from "sick sinus syndrome." These arrhythmias are probably the result of the extensive disturbance of the atrium and the sinus node during the surgical procedures; indeed, some abnormality of rhythm occurs in over half of all children who have undergone these operations, and some of these children may need pacemakers or medication many years after the original operation. Now that most babies with transposition receive arterial switch operations that do not involve surgery in the atrium, arrhythmias are becoming quite unusual.

Arrhythmias following repair of tetralogy of Fallot, on the other hand, are primarily caused by premature ventricular contractions or ventricular tachycardia. These complications are steadily decreasing and it seems very probable that the combination of earlier surgery and newer methods of protecting the myocardium during surgery will make late arrhythmias even less frequent and severe in the future.

Bacterial infections

Bacterial infection can occur as a localized abscess around a stitch in the skin or, occasionally, as an infection of the heart or chest cavity itself. Serious bacterial infection now occurs in fewer than five of one thousand heart operations. Usually the signs of infection, including high fever, develop while the child is still in the hospital, but occasionally the signs are delayed until after the child is discharged. Most such infections can now be treated successfully with large doses of antibiotics and sometimes reopening of the chest.

Viral infections

Viral infections that can affect a child after heart surgery include hepatitis, cytomegalovirus, and AIDS, all caused by infection of the transfused blood used for cardiopulmonary bypass. They are now almost unknown as a consequence of sophisticated blood bank screening techniques. For a brief period, about two years, after the human immunodeficiency virus that causes AIDS became prevalent, a few children did become infected, but this risk has now virtually been abolished.

Postpericardiotomy syndrome

Diane S. was a pretty 4-year-old when she was first found to have an atrial septal defect. Although her doctors recommended surgery to close the defect, Diane was terrified of needles and hospitals, and her mother did not want to force the issue. Her father was not in the home. Eventually, after many conferences with family counselors and the cardiac nurse specialist, Diane agreed to enter the hospital. She was then 7. Repair of the heart defect went smoothly and she went home only six days after surgery, but a week later she felt severe pain under her sternum (breastbone) and when she took a deep breath she felt a stabbing pain in the right side of her chest. Diane and her mother were concerned, even though they had been told about the syndrome; they were worried that the repair was breaking down.

At the heart center the next day the echo test showed fluid around Diane's heart and over her right lung. Once Diane understood that the pain was caused by the two surfaces of the pericardium, or outer lining of the heart, rubbing together, and that it was not coming from inside the heart, she felt better. The fluid disappeared with aspirin treatment. Diane had one more attack of chest pain a year later, but it was a much milder attack than before, and the fluid has not recurred since. She is now about to enter college and is in excellent health.

Accumulation of fluid in and around the heart and lungs, or postpericardiotomy syndrome, is seen only after open-heart operations; it occurs between one and three weeks after surgery. The child develops a low-grade fever and often some pain in the chest. Fluid may accumulate in the pleural cavity surrounding the lungs or in the pericardial cavity around the heart. The problem is thought to be caused by a sensitivity or autoimmune reaction to the surgical opening of the pericardium. There is some evidence also that the reaction involves "lighting up" or reactivation of a preexisting respiratory viral infection. Treatment is with aspirin or a similar medication, such as indomethacin, over a period of from two to four weeks. Readmission to the hospital is needed only if the amount of fluid that has collected by the time of diagnosis is considerable. Rarely, some fluid may need to be removed with a needle. The syndrome is usually little more than a nuisance, a slight blip in an otherwise smooth postoperative course. A few children do experience repeated attacks for a few years, but all such attacks respond to medical treatment, and they do no lasting damage.

This syndrome is much less frequent in infants who undergo surgery before 2 years of age than in older children, perhaps because babies have had less exposure to colds and viral illness.

Neurological damage

Katie C. was born with a very complex heart defect—double outlet right ventricle and coarctation of the aorta. In addition, her left ventricle was hypoplastic. She had emergency surgery as a newborn baby, and at that time the coarctation was repaired and a band was placed on her pulmonary artery to reduce the excessive flow of blood to her lungs and to make the high pressure in her pulmonary artery come down to normal. She stayed on small doses of Lasix to prevent congestion in her lungs, and grew well and started walking and talking.

When she was 3 years old a second operation was performed, in which the veins from the upper part of her body were joined to the pulmonary artery and the band was removed. She looked wonderful the day after surgery, but the next day had a convulsion and was unconscious for several hours. Echo and other tests showed she had some small clots inside her heart. As she recovered, she was left with some weakness in her left arm and leg. Now, at 5 years old, she has had her third operation, a Fontan procedure. For the first time in her life, she is a healthy pink color, and she no longer walks with a limp. She still has less strength in her left hand than in her right, but she is learning to read and write her letters, and the clots that caused the trouble are no longer present. She is a happy, bright child whose family has helped her through all her needed physiotherapy to her remarkable recovery.

Although strokes from clots in the heart may follow surgery, as they did in Katie, strokes can also be a complication in some children who have not had an operation. In a child with a very dilated heart that is beating poorly (dilated cardiomyopathy), small clots may form in the ventricle and shoot off or embolize to the brain, leading to a stroke. This is a serious complication in some children and adults who are awaiting heart transplants. Strokes also used to be a much dreaded complication in severely cyanotic infants with transposition or tetralogy who were awaiting heart surgery. In babies with low oxygen levels in the blood, the blood is thicker than normal and may form deposits in the vessels of the brain, causing a stroke. Now that surgery can be done so early in life, strokes are much rarer in children with heart problems than in the past. One day, we hope, they will no longer occur.

Neurological damage after heart surgery is the most serious of all complications. Even after a very smooth and successful procedure, such as an arterial switch for transposition, seizures may occur in the first two postoperative days. Such seizures are usually easily treated and appear to cause no long-term damage. Stroke occurs after 1 in 400 operations, but recovery is usually complete in such cases.

Profound general neurological damage occurs after one in one thousand operations, usually when surgery has been long and complicated or some intraoperative disaster has occurred, but occasionally, very occasionally, after an apparently uneventful surgical procedure. It is thought that the damage is caused by air or a blood clot that enters the circulation while the child is on the heart-lung machine and reaches the vessels of the brain. The child may be left with some paralysis or even with permanent damage to speech and intelligence. There is no way to write of such tragedies except to say that constant and unremitting effort is devoted to their prevention, and we can only hope that by the time this book is read they will no longer occur.

Bacterial Endocarditis

Because bacterial endocarditis (BE) is a serious disease, the child and the family must take precautions to avoid it. These precautions are called *BE prophylaxis*.

Pedro was a healthy, normal boy who had a loud heart murmur from a small ventricular septal defect, but who kept up with his friends in academics and in sports. When he was 11 he fell while bicycling and cut his knee and his lip. He had slight bleeding from the gums but did not need stitches. About three weeks later he lost his usual healthy appetite and said he had a headache. His pediatrician suspected endocarditis and drew a blood sample. Two days later the laboratory called to say streptococci were growing in the blood sample. Pedro was admitted to the hospital for a week, where his echocardiogram showed no sign of infected clumps (veg-

etations) around the VSD. Once the exact dose of antibiotic he needed was established (this involved several more blood tests), he was allowed to go home and continue with intravenous treatment at home under the supervision of a visiting nurse. Homework was brought to him while he was out of school; he was off all medication, had returned to full activity, and was back in his regular classroom five weeks after the illness started.

Like most other conditions we have talked about in this book, endocarditis shows a wide spectrum of severity, and not all children can be treated at home during part of the illness. Complications of endocarditis still occur; these include stroke caused by infected clots that break off from the valve or site of infection and heart-valve damage caused by spread of the infection (as happened in Ronnie L., whose story is told in chapter 12).

Endocarditis is a bacterial infection of the endocardium, the inner lining of the heart wall. Families and professionals find discussion of preventing endocarditis difficult. For one thing, no one has come up with a brief phrase consisting of short, common words to describe the methods of prevention. We use the phrase *BE prophylaxis* (*prophylaxis*, Greek, prevention) in this book, but no one can say it rolls trippingly off the tongue.

Endocarditis begins with a fever and sometimes with some small spots under the skin (*petechiae*). It can be caused by almost any bacterium, but the streptococcus and staphylococcus are usually responsible. If a child with a heart defect runs a fever without any obvious cause for three days or longer, the physician will search for signs of petechiae. Even if they are absent, the physician may arrange for a blood culture, since finding bacteria in the bloodstream is the only certain method of diagnosis. An echocardiogram is sometimes helpful in showing whether there are large clumps of bacteria and clots attached to part of the heart, but if the disease is diagnosed early there may be no echocardiographic changes. Before the days of antibiotics, endocarditis led to a long debilitating illness with loss of weight, anemia, an enlarged spleen, and often a number of changes in the skin, the urine, and the nail beds. Cures were rare. Diagnosis is now usually made early and treatment is successful more than 80 percent of the time. When endocarditis occurs in a small premature baby as a complication of prolonged intravenous feeding, or when it is caused by bacteria injected with unsterile needles into the bloodstream by a drug abuser, treatment is particularly difficult.

> *Why does Jane need to take amoxicillin when she goes to the dentist? She's on the swim team and is more active than her brother Jerry. I know Jane has a small ventricular septal defect. They told me it would never trouble her, so why does she need to worry about endocarditis?*

In many heart defects, including VSD, a turbulent eddy of blood flows around the child's heart defect; bacteria circulating in the bloodstream may move into this eddy and infect the site of the defect. Very few, if any, bacteria usually circulate through the heart; however, bacteria can be released from the mouth and reach the heart through the bloodstream during major dental work or other manipulations involving bleeding from the gums.

If preventive measures such as the use of amoxicillin are necessary for the child, the family (and the growing child) should carry one of the American Heart Association cards describing the correct timing and dosage of medications and the name of the cardiologist or primary physician to call with questions (see figure 14.1).

> *Does everyone with a heart murmur need to take amoxicillin for all dental procedures?*

No, it depends on whether the murmur is caused by a jet of blood going through a narrow opening: such a jet causes turbulent flow and makes endocarditis more likely. Your physician will be able to decide whether this precaution is necessary.

> *Why do some children need to go on taking precautions even after heart surgery, while others don't?*

The nature of the heart problem makes the difference: for example, after surgery on the aortic valve, the valve is still thick and endocarditis is possible. But after a patent ductus has been repaired, prophylaxis is no longer needed.

> *How great is the risk of endocarditis?*

Fortunately the risk is continually decreasing, partly because children's teeth are now so well cared for and partly because nowadays many heart defects are repaired in infancy. Children at high risk in-

Name: _____

needs protection from
BACTERIAL ENDOCARDITIS
because of an existing
HEART CONDITION

Diagnosis: _____

Prescribed by: _____

Date: _____

For Dental/Oral/Upper Respiratory Tract Procedures

I. Standard Regimen In Patients At Risk (includes those with prosthetic heart valves and other high risk patients):

Amoxicillin 3.0 g orally one hour before procedure, then 1.5 g six hours after initial dose.*

For amoxicillin/penicillin-allergic patients:

Erythromycin ethylsuccinate 800 mg or erythromycin stearate 1.0 g orally 2 hours before a procedure, then one-half the dose 6 hours after the initial administration.*

—OR—

Clindamycin 300 mg orally 1 hour before a procedure and 150 mg 6 hours after initial dose.*

II. Alternate Prophylactic Regimens For Dental/Oral/Upper Respiratory Tract Procedures In Patients At Risk:

A. For patients unable to take oral medications:

Ampicillin 2.0 g IV (or IM) 30 minutes before procedure, then ampicillin 1.0 g IV (or IM) OR amoxicillin 1.5 g orally 6 hours after initial dose.*

—OR—

For ampicillin/amoxicillin/penicillin-allergic patients unable to take oral medications:

Clindamycin 300 mg IV 30 minutes before a procedure and 150 mg IV (or orally) 6 hours after initial dose.*

B. For patients considered to be at high risk who are not candidates for the standard regimen:

Ampicillin 2.0 g IV (or IM) plus gentamicin 1.5 mg/kg IV (or IM) (not to exceed 80 mg) 30 minutes before procedure, followed by amoxicillin 1.5 g orally 6 hours after the initial dose. Alternatively, the parenteral regimen may be repeated 8 hours after the initial dose.*

For amoxicillin/ampicillin/penicillin-allergic patients considered to be at high risk:

Vancomycin 1.0 g IV administered over one hour, starting one hour before the procedure. No repeat dose is necessary.*

*Note: Initial pediatric dosages are listed below. Follow-up oral dose should be one-half the inital dose. Total pediatric dose should not exceed total adult dose.

Amoxicillin:†	50 mg/kg	Vancomycin:	20 mg/kg
Clindamycin:	10 mg/kg	Ampicillin:	50 mg/kg
Erythromycin ethylsuccinate		Gentamicin:	2.0 mg/kg
or stearate:	20 mg/kg		

† The following weight ranges may also be used for the initial pediatric dose of amoxicillin:
<15 kg (33 lbs), 750 mg
15–30 kg (33–66 lbs), 1500 mg
>30 kg (66 lbs), 3000 mg (full adult dose)

Kilogram to pound conversion chart: (1 kg = 2.2 lb)

Kg	Lb
5	11.0
10	22.0
20	44.0
30	66.0
40	88.0
50	110.0

For Genitourinary/Gastrointestinal Procedures

I. Standard regimen:

Ampicillin 2.0 g IV (or IM) plus gentamicin 1.5 mg/kg IV (or IM) (not to exceed 80 mg) 30 minutes before procedure, followed by amoxicillin 1.5 g orally 6 hours after the initial dose. Alternatively, the parenteral regimen may be repeated once 8 hours after the initial dose.*

For amoxicillin/ampicillin/penicillin-allergic patients:

Vancomycin 1.0 g IV administered over 1 hour plus gentamicin 1.5 mg/kg IV (or IM) (not to exceed 80 mg) one hour before the procedure. May be repeated once 8 hours after initial dose.**

II. Alternate oral regimen for low-risk patients:

Amoxicillin 3.0 g orally one hour before the procedure, then 1.5 g 6 hours after the initial dose.**

** Note: Initial pediatric dosages are listed below. Follow-up oral dose should be one-half the initial dose. Total pediatric dose should not exceed total adult dose.

Ampicillin:	50 mg/kg	Gentamicin:	2.0 mg/kg
Amoxicillin:	50 mg/kg	Vancomycin:	20 mg/kg

Note: Antibiotic regimens used to prevent recurrences of acute rheumatic fever are inadequate for the prevention of bacterial endocarditis. In patients with markedly compromised renal function, it may be necessary to modify or omit the second dose of gentamicin or vancomycin. Intramuscular injections may be contraindicated in patients receiving anticoagulants.

Adapted from *Prevention of Bacterial Endocarditis: Recommendations by the American Heart Association* by the Committee on Rheumatic Fever, Endocarditis, and Kawasaki Disease. *JAMA* 1990;264:2919–2922, © 1990 American Medical Association (also excerpted in *J Am Dent Assoc* 1991;122:87–92).

Please refer to these joint American Heart Association–American Dental Association recommendations for more complete information as to which patients and which procedures require prophylaxis.

♥ American Heart Association

National Center
7320 Greenville Avenue
Dallas, Texas 75231

78-1003 (CP)
90-91-611.2M
6-91-890M
90 06 19 B   ♻ printed on recycled paper

The Council on Dental Therapeutics of the American Dental Association has approved this statement as it relates to dentistry.

14.1. Bacterial Endocarditis Card, 1990. Reproduced with permission. Copyright American Heart Association.

clude those with artificial valves in their hearts. In a large cardiac center that treats more than three thousand children with heart problems annually, only two children out of the three thousand will have endocarditis. Endocarditis is a serious disease; prevention is the goal.

Can it always be prevented?

No. Sometimes there is no recognizable source of infection, however carefully we look. That is why it is important to be aware of the early signs: *fever* without an obvious cause that lasts more than three days; *fatigue* with loss of energy and the usual childhood joie de vivre; *loss of appetite*; and a *pallid appearance*.

The Risk of Complications

Complications of heart problems depend on what exactly is wrong with the heart and how the heart problem affects the other parts of the body. Endocarditis can complicate a ventricular septal defect, even a very small one, but only large ventricular septal defects cause the complication of heart failure with congestion of the lungs and the liver and delay in growth. The prevention of complications, and their early recognition and effective treatment, are important topics to be discussed as soon as a heart problem is recognized. The risk of some complications becomes much lower after surgery. For example, someone with a ventricular septal defect that has not been corrected through surgery has a 12-percent risk of developing endocarditis at some time during a normal life span, but after the defect is completely closed, either by natural closure or by surgery, the risk is almost zero.

Of course, treatment of any kind can lead to complications, and before any cardiac medication is started the risks and benefits need to be reviewed by the family and health team. Because surgery is so successful in most children, long-term medication is seldom necessary. When medications are prescribed, the family must be aware of any possible side effects, and what to do if they occur. Complications from medications used to treat heart failure or arrhythmias can occur in about one in ten infants and children with such conditions, but they are almost invariably short-lived and treatable.

Complications of surgery may result in damage to the heart itself or to nearby structures such as nerves or lymph vessels. Or complications may arise from an infection or an autoimmune reaction to the opening up of the pericardium and heart muscle. The incidence of complications varies from 1 percent or less for complications following ductus ligation to a very high rate of 50 percent or more for arrhythmias that follow atrial operations for transposition.

A steady and dramatic decrease in complications from all types of treatment has accompanied the movement toward early surgery and our improved understanding of how the myocardium functions and how its wonderful force of contraction can be preserved.

Chapter 15

Children with Multiple Handicaps

The fact that a child has a heart problem does not usually mean that the child has a lot of other difficulties. Sometimes, if an atrial septal defect is recognized for the first time after infancy is past, say in a 5-year-old child, parents may ask themselves, "What are they going to find next? What else is wrong that we don't know about?" This is a time when it is reassuring to remember that three in four heart defects occur in children who are otherwise entirely healthy, with normal intelligence and no abnormality in any other part of the body. Although some transient disturbance affected the flow of blood through the heart at a critical moment during fetal development and the atrial septum did not close as it should, everything else was formed perfectly.

About one in four children born with a heart defect has an abnormality elsewhere in the body. A child may be born with a heart defect and mental retardation, or there may be defects in other organs as well as in the heart. These defects may be too mild to cause delays in growth and development, or they may be serious enough to interfere with normal growth and living.

In general, children who have certain heart defects are more likely than others to have multiple handicaps. A child with an atrial septal defect, transposition, or pulmonic stenosis, for example, only rarely has any problems outside the heart itself. Or if there is a problem it is something like a hernia, an extra fifth finger, or webbing between the toes—a relatively trivial problem that runs in the family or ethnic group and is quite unrelated to the heart.

But children who have endocardial cushion defects, interrupted aortic arch, or tetralogy of Fallot more often have other real problems. For some of these children the heart may be the major problem; in others several handicapping conditions co-exist and interact with each other, making prolonged and complicated treatment plans necessary. To take a simple example, a baby girl who has both tetralogy of Fallot and a cleft palate will need more operations in infancy, and more special feeding methods; she will have an increased risk of ear infections, and later on she will need speech therapy. This child may emerge as a happy and nearly normal child, but the stress for her and her parents will clearly be greater than if tetralogy was her only problem.

Syndromes That Often Have Heart Problems Associated with Them

While some heart defects are usually isolated, others almost always occur as part of a syndrome. For example, the form of endocardial cushion defect known as a complete atrioventricular canal is commonly associated with Down syndrome (trisomy 21). (See Rachel's story in this chapter.)

The following list includes some of the other syndromes commonly associated with heart defects. "AD" and "AR" refer to the autosomal dominant and autosomal recessive modes of inheritance.

- Allagille: The baby with Allagille syndrome has an abnormal liver with fibrosis of the biliary ducts, leading to jaundice, itching, and slow growth; the heart defect is peripheral pulmonary stenosis. Genetics variable; some AD.
- Beckwith-Wiedemann: The liver is large, the blood sugar is low, and the heart muscle is thickened (hypertrophic cardiomyopathy). Some AD; some have abnormal chromosome 11p.
- *CHARGE*: The cornea of the eye may be incomplete (*C*oloboma), the *H*eart defect is usually ventricular septal defect or tetralogy; there is blockage of one nostril (choanal *A*tresia), there is a kidney (*R*enal) and *G*enital abnormality; the child has cup-shaped *E*ars and deafness. Sporadic, that is, cause unknown; does not run in family.
- Di George: The thymus gland may be small or absent, causing problems with the immune system that may lead to low resistance to infection and abnormal response to blood transfu-

sions. The parathyroid glands also may be defective, leading to low levels of calcium in the blood. The heart problem is usually a truncus, interrupted aortic arch, or tetralogy of Fallot with pulmonary atresia. Genetics: may be AD or AR; some babies are missing part of chromosome 22. The syndrome may be sporadic or may follow acutane use before or during pregnancy.

- Down (trisomy 21): The most frequent and so the most important of these syndromes; see Rachel's story in this chapter.

- Ehlers-Danlos: Ehlers-Danlos syndrome is a connective tissue disorder, meaning that the skin and joints are less firm than usual and have less elastic properties; the skin is loose, the joints bend into abnormal positions, and easy bruising occurs. Mitral valve prolapse is the most usual heart problem. Genetics: usually AR.

- Ellis van Creveld: Ellis van Creveld syndrome is a rare form of dwarfism. The baby has polydactyly (too many fingers and toes); is very short, with abnormal cartilage at the ends of the bones; and characteristically has a very large atrial septal defect (single atrium, a type of endocardial cushion defect). Genetics: AR; clusters are seen in Amish communities. Repair of the heart defect will not make the child grow, but is nevertheless usually needed to avoid heart failure.

- Facio-Velar-Cardiac: See Shprintzen.

- Fanconi: This is a very rare syndrome, with difficulty in chromosome repair. The baby has small thumbs, often a brownish discoloration of the skin, and a ventricular septal defect. The life-threatening problem is severe anemia; other blood disorders, including leukemia, are often present. Genetics: AR.

- Fetal Alcohol: In severely affected babies the face is abnormal in shape, the fingers are short and stubby, and the intelligence is low; learning disability is a major problem. A variety of heart defects may occur, the most common of which are atrial or ventricular septal defects.

- Glycogen storage: There are several familial syndromes that involve defects in the breakdown of glycogen to glucose and may cause cardiomyopathy by a buildup of glycogen in the heart. See Pompé syndrome.

- Goldenhaar: One side of the face is smaller than the other. There may be a skin tag in front of the ear, deafness, and a missing area in the cornea of the eye (coloboma). Heart defects are present in one of three children with the syndrome and may include tetralogy of Fallot. Genetics: usually sporadic, that is, no family pattern, but sometimes AD.

- Holt-Oram: Holt-Oram was originally described as an AD syndrome with absent thumb and an atrial septal defect. Abnormalities of the radius (forearm bone) may lead to finger-like (digitalized) thumb or a severe arm defect. Cardiac defects vary, but they usually involve septation; atrial septal defects are most frequent.

- Hypertrophic cardiomyopathy: Usually children with this AD disorder have no defects outside the heart. Some have many pigmented moles (lentigenes) and the term LEOPARD syndrome may be used for the occurrence in combination of Lentigenes, EKG abnormalities, Ocular change (eyes wide apart), Pulmonary stenosis, Abnormal genital organs, Retardation, and Deafness. It is likely that this syndrome is closely related to neurofibromatosis and may overlap with Noonan-Ehmke.

- Ivemark: Ivemark syndrome is a useful inclusive term for disorders of looping associated with asplenia or polysplenia. Since Ivemark first described the complex heart defects seen in such infants, a great deal has been learned about early recognition and treatment. Babies born without a spleen (asplenia) usually have large endocardial cushion defects and also transposition and abnormal pulmonary veins. Babies with several spleens (polysplenia) have fewer severe heart problems, usually a septal defect and pulmonary stenosis. Genetics: probably AR, but fewer than one in four siblings is affected.

- Kartagener: There is a defect in the movement of the cilia that help to move secretions; the nasal sinuses are blocked, the lungs may be chronically infected, and males are usually sterile. Dextrocardia of the mirror image type, without other heart defects, is frequent. Genetics: AR. Both Ivemark and Kartagener have occurred in some families.

- Marfan: Tall stature and long fingers and toes are associated with eye abnormalities (dislocated lens) and skeletal problems including scoliosis (spinal curvature) and a narrow chest (pectus). The heart shows mitral valve prolapse and the aorta gets progressively larger as the child grows. Careful follow-up of the heart is needed. Genetics: mostly AD, but some of the most severely affected children are sporadic (have no family history) and have a spontaneous mutation. Recent studies by Dr. Hal Dietz and colleagues at Johns Hopkins have localized the defect to a gene on chromosome 15 involved in making fibrillin, which is part of normal connective tissue.

- Mucopolysaccharoidosis: In Hurler syndrome, the most common type of mucopolysaccharoidosis, abnormal deposits of a protein in cartilage, brain, and heart lead to a coarsening of facial features, stunting of growth, and thickening of the heart valves as the child grows. Genetics: varies with different subgroups; Hurler is AR.

- Muscular Dystrophies: In the Duchenne type, the most common of the muscular dystrophies in children, there is a defect in muscle protein due to a defective dystrophin gene. This defect leads to increasing muscle weakness, often complicated by cardiomyopathy. Genetics: varies; Duchenne affects boys, but the defective gene is carried by the mother (sex-linked recessive).

- Noonan-Ehmke: Noonan-Ehmke syndrome is characterized by short stature with wide-apart eyes, a tendency to form spread-out keloid scars, varying degrees of mental retardation, and pulmonary stenosis due to a thickened dysplastic pulmonary valve. Genetics: AD; some mildly affected family members may be undiagnosed for many years. A point-scoring system devised by Duncan is helpful in deciding if the syndrome is present; no laboratory test is yet available.

- Osteogenesis imperfecta: The bones are fragile and easily fractured. In the heart the aorta may be dilated, with aortic valve insufficiency. Different genetic types; AR most frequent.

- Pompé: Pompé syndrome involves an inherited deficiency in the enzyme alpha 1 maltase, leading to accumulation of glycogen in the muscles and the heart. It is the worst form of glycogen storage disease of the heart and an example of a genetic (AR) form of metabolic cardiomyopathy.

- Long QT: The long QT syndrome is a disorder of the nervous system control of the heart, resulting in a prolonged interval between the Q wave and T wave on the electrocardiogram and tendency to develop severe arrhythmia (ventricular tachycardia or **fibrillation**) during stress or exercise. Usually the child is otherwise normal (Romano Ward Syndrome) and inheritance is AD; when there is also familial deafness (Jervell Lange Nielson syndrome), inheritance is AR.

- Rubella: If the mother has German measles (rubella) in early pregnancy, the infant may have congenital deafness, cataracts, and sometimes mental retardation. Patent ductus and pulmonary arterial stenosis are the most usual heart problems. This is a preventable "environmental" defect, not a genetic syndrome.

- Scimitar: The right lung and pulmonary artery are small, and the right pulmonary veins form an unusual scimitar-shaped shadow on chest X-ray as they drain into the inferior caval vein. Some children have large arteries from the aorta supplying the right lung and others have additional defects of the urinary tract. Sometimes familial (AD), but usually does not run in family.

- Shprintzen: The palate shows a high arch or cleft, and speech difficulty is associated with either a ventricular septal defect or tetralogy of Fallot. Probably AD.

- Smith-Lemli-Opitz: Mental retardation and a small head (microcephaly) are associated with abnormal fingers and toes and various heart defects including atrial and ventricular septal defects and tetralogy. Genetics: AR.

- *TAR* (thrombocytopenia absent radius): This syndrome involves a severe defect of both arms, accompanied by low **platelets** in the circulating blood. Bleeding may be a serious problem. The heart defect is usually an atrial septal defect or tetralogy. Genetics: AR.

- Trisomies 13 and 18: Babies with trisomy 13 or 18 have much worse mental retardation and many more deformities than those with trisomy 21 (Down syndrome). Heart defects are nearly always present but are overshadowed by the other problems.

- Turner (*XO*): Girls with Turner syndrome have only one X chromosome and their ovaries do not function. Left heart flow defects are usual, varying from hypoplastic left heart ventricle to bicuspid aortic valve.

- *VACTERL*: VACTERL syndrome is characterized by Vertebral, Anal, Cardiac, Tracheo-esophageal, Renal, and Limb abnormalities. Genetics: usually sporadic, sometimes seen with maternal diabetes. Heart defect is usually ventricular septal defect, sometimes tetralogy.

- Williams': An infant with Williams' syndrome may have high levels of calcium in the blood, severe feeding difficulty and irritability, and a small "elfin" face. Older children have thicker features, varying degrees of mental retardation, and abnormal teeth. The heart shows supravalvar aortic and pulmonary narrowing. Genetics: probably AD, although some appear sporadic. It is unclear whether an abnormal genetic response to calcium is involved.

- X-linked cardiomyopathy: Some infants with this syndrome have cataracts and severe retardation associated with thickening of the myocardium, all due to a defect on the X chromosome.

The *"Tower of Babel" syndrome* is not an official term used in textbooks, but it can sometimes be shorthand for the conflicting stories parents receive if multiple experts are seeing their baby. It is very important for any baby with a syndrome to have an ombudsman, a member of the health care team who is looking at the whole picture and helping the family understand what is going on.

Down Syndrome and a Heart Defect

Rachel M. was the second baby born to a healthy young couple. Her mother was 23, her father 25. No one in either family had been born with any defects. The mother experienced a normal pregnancy, although she said Rachel had been less active in the womb than her brother, Joshua, had been. At birth Rachel weighed five pounds, ten ounces, a little underweight. Her facial appearance, the creases in the palms of her hands, the irises of her eyes, and several other findings suggested Down syndrome. Her pediatrician performed a complete physical and concluded that chromosome studies were needed. Noting a soft heart murmur, he also recommended an EKG and an echo-Doppler test. Rachel's parents were tremendously upset to learn that she had Down syndrome; they had thought this was a risk only if the mother was 35 or older. The physician explained that Down syndrome babies can be born to parents of any age; further, he told Rachel's parents that almost half of all babies who have Down syndrome also have heart defects. It was important, the physician told them, to determine whether Rachel did, so that a good plan could be developed to help her.

Rachel's parents were partially correct; Down syndrome does occur more frequently in the babies of older mothers, but it is not only older mothers who are at risk. Unfortunately, the widespread publicity given to the increased risk for older mothers has obscured the fact that most infants with Down syndrome are born to women under the age of 30. Nor can the syndrome always be detected in the fetus. Rachel's mother had had an ultrasound test at twenty-two weeks, but no abnormality had been detected. The signs of Down syndrome on ultrasound are rather subtle, and rarely lead to diagnosis unless suspicion is already high and other tests are done. A relatively new test, the alpha fetoprotein test, which can be done early in pregnancy, promises to be useful as a clue that Down syndrome may be present; the mother can then consider amniocentesis, which would show conclusively whether the fetus's chromosomes are normal or not. If Down syndrome is confirmed early enough, the parents can decide whether or not to continue the pregnancy.

By the time Rachel and her mother went home together four days later, Rachel was feeding well. The chromosome results were not yet back, but the cardiologist had diagnosed a complete atrioventricular canal defect. She had explained the nature of this heart problem to Rachel's parents. Surgical repair would be needed before Rachel's first birthday, probably at around 6 months. No heart medications were needed at present. The cardiologist had arranged to meet with the pediatrician and the parents the evening before Rachel went home: they all looked at the echo-Doppler test and the booklet explaining the test. This meeting was very useful; later, at home, the family talked over many questions. Their sense of shared information was a bond in a very difficult time.

Rachel's parents learned about the many possible handicaps Rachel could face as a consequence of Down syndrome:

• Abnormal facial appearance
• Delayed growth

- Mental retardation
- Risk of other childhood problems, including low thyroid hormone levels in blood (hypothyroidism) and frequent infections
- Skeletal weakness, especially in the hip and the atlanto-axial joint of the neck
- Blood disorders, including increased risk of leukemia
- Possible risk of early onset of Alzheimer's disease

Several things helped Rachel's family in this time of great stress. The pediatrician had a particular interest in Down syndrome and spent considerable time talking with Rachel's parents about her present and future, emphasizing in particular how modern approaches, such as infant stimulation programs, could greatly improve her floppy muscle tone. He stressed the advantages of enrolling Rachel in a Down syndrome center and recommended that the family join the active local support group for parents of similar children.

When Rachel went home from the nursery it was already clear that she did not have some of the other defects known to occur sometimes in Down syndrome, such as obstruction of the intestine (duodenal stenosis or atresia) or dislocated hips. Nevertheless, she would need a heart catheter test at about 2 months and her heart defect would have to be repaired before she was 6 months old.

As all parents know, children do not always follow the pathways laid out for them, and this proved to be the case with Rachel.

> Rachel continued to be a "floppy" baby and fed much more slowly than her brother, Joshua, had done. She was growing slowly, and was a little behind on the Down syndrome growth chart. At 2 months old, before the heart catheter test had been done, she developed her fourth respiratory infection, which rapidly developed almost overnight into severe wheezing and labored breathing. Rachel was admitted to the pediatric intensive care unit. She was found to have a viral infection (respiratory syncytial virus), and treatment with an antiviral agent (Ribavirin) was prescribed. After a critical illness of a few days, Rachel slowly recovered and went home.
>
> At home, Rachel tired more easily than before and when she lay on her back her breathing was loud and snorting. The pediatrician, the cardiologist, and a specialist in children's ear problems concluded that her adenoids, which had grown so large that they were obstructing her breathing and putting an extra strain on her

heart, would have to be removed before she could safely have anes-
thesia for her heart defect.

Rachel's atrioventricular canal defect was repaired when she
was 7 months old. She was in the hospital for eight days and in the
three years that followed, she had no complications and needed no
heart medications. She does have tubes in both ears because of fre-
quent ear problems, and she receives medication for hypothy-
roidism. Rachel is in an infant stimulation program and is starting
nursery school.

Because Rachel's nose and throat passages were narrow, any growth of adenoids or tonsils was likely to block her breathing more than it might in another child. Her heart defect made her lungs congested and more at risk of severe viral infection than the lungs of other babies of her age. Any interference with her breathing put more of a strain on her heart than it would have if her heart had been a healthy one. With her heart defect repaired many of her handicaps are gone, but some will be with her all her life. Mental retardation will be her most serious handicap.

Although the heart defect is not always the child's most severe handicap, its exact nature and effects must be defined. In Rachel this was not difficult, because the atrioventricular canal defect was recognized early; it was a serious defect requiring early repair, but there was an excellent chance of a good surgical result. Without repair, heart failure, poor growth, and possibly development of high pressure in the lungs and damage to the lung arteries can result. This damage to the lung arteries, called the "Eisenmenger reaction," is now rare. (Its effects are described in the story of Edwin later in this chapter.) In this case, a decision in favor of early aggressive treatment is relatively easy.

It is much more difficult to predict how the other problems of Down syndrome will affect a child like Rachel. All children with Down syndrome show delayed mental and physical development, but the severity of the mental retardation varies. The family needs to learn how to help such children reach their best potential, and to plan ahead to prevent any secondary handicaps, such as those caused by hypothyroidism.

The stresses faced by Rachel and her parents during her turbulent early months cannot be exaggerated. In past years few infants born with both Down syndrome and a heart defect survived beyond their first birthday. In the few who did, the effects of high pressure in the lungs became apparent after a period of six to twelve years. With a complete atrioventricular canal defect, like Rachel's, the pressure in the lungs is high as a result of the large defect in the center of the heart (figure 6.1). Gradually the small arteries in the lungs (**arterioles**) become damaged by this high pressure; their walls thicken and let less and less blood through. Eventually blood flow to the lungs becomes so obstructed that blood begins to go from the *right to the left side* of the heart through the defect (instead of from left to right), and the child becomes blue (cyanotic). This is the Eisenmenger reaction. Early in this century it was reported that some children who had not been blue in infancy did become blue later (*cyanose tardive*, or delayed cyanosis). It was not then understood how the heart and lungs act upon each other. Some adults who have Down syndrome have this additional handicap of severe cyanosis, but surgery is not possible for them because their lung arterioles are now so badly blocked.

> *Edwin is 29. His mother was 37 when he was born. He was thought to look abnormal at birth, but the diagnosis of Down syndrome was not made until he was 6 months old. He had a heart murmur, and his growth as a baby was slow and he had frequent respiratory infections. He went to a special school and slowly learned to say a few words.*
>
> *At the age of 3 Edwin saw a cardiologist, who suspected an atrioventricular canal defect with severe damage to the arteries in the lungs. A cardiac catheter test confirmed this suspicion, but it was already too late to repair Edwin's heart. At 7 years he became blue (cyanotic) when he exercised, but not until he was 18 did he begin to have the bad headaches attributed to his cyanosis. His headaches and shortness of breath eased after he had some blood removed.*

This periodic removal of one or two pints of blood, now called *phlebotomy* (once described as "bloodletting"), is used in an occasional adult like Edwin to reduce the number of red blood cells circulating. The mass of the red cells is increased in response to the low oxygen level in the blood—an increase in red cells that is useful, up to a certain point, because they carry more oxygen. After that point, however, a sort of "overshoot" occurs, the blood becomes thick and viscous, almost treacly, and tends to clot in the small arteries of the lungs and in the brain. When this occurs, phlebotomy (and, often, half an aspirin tablet a day) is recommended to prevent stroke and further lung damage.

Edwin continues to have phlebotomy about every six weeks as an outpatient. In the last five years, he has been in the hospital three times for short periods for heart failure.

Edwin's mother, a practical nurse, has helped to make him a real member of the family. On most days he goes to a sheltered workshop. His mother administers his cardiac medications; oxygen is available for his use at night if he needs it.

Edwin's late cyanosis was a consequence of the Eisenmenger reaction. Now that early repair of atrioventricular canal defects is done in infancy, other children in the United States will not experience a similar series of problems. In some other countries where early repair is not done, however, children like Edwin will continue to reach adulthood burdened with the handicaps with which they were born and with new ones.

Other Multiple Handicaps

Doctors have less experience with other multiple handicaps than with Down syndrome; therefore, treatment of children with multiple handicaps is often delayed and its effects on the child are less predictable.

Noonan-Ehmke syndrome

Glenn B. was born weighing four pounds, five ounces. His mother had a normal pregnancy. She had always been healthy, and she had a daughter, now 4, who was entirely normal. Soon after Glenn's birth, the pediatrician heard a loud heart murmur over Glenn's chest and told the parents that Glenn had pulmonary stenosis and might need early surgery. Glenn grew very slowly, and after a catheter test confirmed severe pulmonary stenosis, surgery was done. The pulmonary valve was found to be thick and "dysplastic"; part of it was removed to relieve the obstruction.

Glenn grew just as slowly after the operation as he had before; it became apparent that he was not sitting up or standing at the same age at which his sister had. He was 18 months old before it was recognized that both he and his mother had Noonan-Ehmke syndrome. He has remained a slow learner, but nevertheless has graduated from high school and is now working. He and his mother and a younger brother, who also has the syndrome, are all active in the Little People of America organization.

Noonan-Ehmke syndrome is an example of a combination of handicaps that may not be fully recognized at birth. Sometimes undue early attention is focused on the heart and the family believes, mistakenly, that the child will be completely normal once heart surgery is done. Noonan-Ehmke syndrome is characterized by short stature, eyes that are set wide apart, varying degrees of mental retardation, a tendency to form wide keloid scars, and pulmonary stenosis. When the pulmonary valve is stenotic, it is usually thick and dysplastic (badly formed), as it was in Glenn, and cannot be treated by balloon valvuloplasty. The syndrome is inherited in an autosomal dominant mode (see chapter 3), meaning that Mrs. B. and others like her have almost a fifty-fifty chance of transmitting the condition to a child, regardless of the other parent's genetic makeup. Mildly affected family members may be undiagnosed for years. Glenn's mother was quite short (under five feet), but this fact alone did not immediately alert the medical staff.

In some children there is no clue in early infancy that any handicap exists except in the heart itself.

Tetralogy with pulmonary atresia and a speech defect

Diane G. was a twin, weighing three pounds at birth; she was intensely blue immediately after birth and was found to have tetralogy with pulmonary atresia. Her twin sister was healthy. After two shunt operations, Diane had open-heart repair of her heart defect at a heart center far from her home. Her pulmonary valve and artery were replaced. Although she was still small (seven pounds) when this surgery was done, the operation was successful; Diane became a normal pink color, began to grow, and became very active, although she was always smaller than her twin.

By 28 months, however, Diane was not talking at all, although in every other way she was clearly a very bright child. After many tests it was discovered that she had been born with a defect in the speech center in her brain. She has now made excellent progress with speech therapy.

Diane's parents had already been through a great deal before they became aware that she had a combination of handicaps that were not obvious at the time of her birth. They helped Diane face this new hurdle with the same courage and persistence they had shown in the anxious times of her early heart surgery. They have remained a close and loving family.

It is clearer now than it was when Diane was born that infants with tetralogy and pulmonary atresia are especially likely to have other problems outside the heart. Often the problem involves part of the nervous system, as it did in Diane, or other tissues that developed from the neural crest cells that help form the conotruncal area of the heart.

- Each handicapping condition has its own effect; usually the heart defect and any mental handicap are the most serious.
- Defects may interact: for example, if a baby has a VACTERL syndrome, with numerous abnormalities, speech may be delayed by a cleft palate, by repeated ear infections and resulting deafness, and by the prolonged hospital stays to treat the infections. The degree of speech delay may be more severe than would be expected on the basis of other tests of intelligence and development.
- A specialist in each particular problem, sometimes a geneticist or a cardiologist, can help predict future effects of that problem and can contribute to an overall plan.

One of the special problems of children with multiple handicaps is the correct interpretation of the meaning of symptoms. Even in these days of high-technology medicine, interpretation can be a challenge.

Despite severe problems, a child who has multiple handicaps may bring happiness and courage and a new insight into life to the family and to the health team.

Severe retardation and tetralogy

Debbie B. was born with trisomy 13 (a syndrome characterized by severe mental retardation and numerous deformities, usually including defects in the heart) and tetralogy of Fallot. Her parents learned that her life expectancy was short; they were determined to give her the best possible care during the time she had. They joined a trisomy support group and received a great deal of help.

At about 6 months of age Debbie began to have severe episodes ("blue spells") in which she turned blue and became limp. She seemed to be in pain during these attacks, which were attributed to her heart. After considerable discussion, it was decided to perform a shunt operation to improve blood flow to her lungs. The oxygen level in her blood improved, but the spells were no better than they had been before surgery. More tests showed that Debbie was "aspi-

*rating," that is, that much of her food was going into her lungs
rather than into her stomach. A Nissen procedure, a stomach operation that is usually successful for aspiration, was performed, but
it did not help, and Debbie died about six weeks later. She had
spent the last two months of her short life in the hospital. The consolation of the family and her health team was that they did all
they could.*

This story illustrates how very difficult it can sometimes be to follow the "right" course in cases where many handicaps interact. Debbie
showed us that even in the best of circumstances it may be hard to
know which problem is causing the effect we see. In retrospect, it
seems likely that Debbie's "blue spells" were caused more by a severe
nervous system defect, which also led to continuous aspiration, than by
any treatable problem in her lungs or her esophagus.

Treatments and Decisions

In some infants it is clear at birth that one problem is present (in
Rachel's case, it was Down syndrome), and a diligent search is made for
other problems known to be frequent in such children. In other infants, a heart defect is recognized at once, but an associated mental retardation or other handicap comes to notice only later. Very few full-
term babies who appear active and vigorous at birth except for signs of
a heart difficulty are found to have an additional major problem. But in
babies of low birth weight who are very slow to cry and move, and who
have abnormalities of the face, additional severe handicaps must always
be suspected.

The type of heart defect is also a clue to the presence of other
handicaps. For example, two out of three babies who have endocardial
cushion defects also have other major handicaps, almost always Down
syndrome. By contrast, one in ten babies with hypoplastic right ventricle also has another defect, and only rarely does such an infant have
abnormalities of the chromosomes.

In a few infants, the child's heart problem progresses during childhood and adolescence. For example, in Marfan syndrome, which is
characterized by various abnormalities, careful follow-up of the heart
will be needed because the aorta becomes progressively larger as the
child grows.

Depending on the individual child and the heart defect present, cardiac care may be critically important throughout childhood; increasingly, the heart defect can be corrected early. Cardiac checkups may continue, but the principal focus after infancy will be coordination of a child's educational and developmental needs.

After the multiple handicaps are identified, a treatment plan is developed. The plan cannot be generalized, for each child is different. Whenever possible, a specialist should be asked to help resolve the most urgent issues to be faced and to guide the family to see the future in as realistic and as positive a way as possible. Support groups are of great value; some provide informative newsletters and arrange useful meetings. Support groups exist for families of infants with Williams' and Down syndromes and with various forms of glycogen storage disease.

The federal government has developed a new program to organize a special center in every state to coordinate the care of infants and children at high risk of delayed development. This new program is already proving to be a major advance. In Maryland it is called the Maryland Infants and Toddlers Program, and all the agencies work together to help a child with multiple handicaps.

Of some infants born with severe multiple handicaps the question is sometimes asked, Should anything be done except to provide nourishment and compassionate care? This agonizing question is sometimes termed an "ethical" one, as if ethics were somehow separate from all medicine and child care. The answer is that rarely, when an infant's life expectancy with or without treatment is clearly less than two years, it may be appropriate to consider withholding cardiac or other technologically advanced care. More than one meeting between the health team and the family may be needed before a decision can be reached. Very occasionally, when resolution of the problem is particularly difficult, the involvement of someone from the hospital ethics committee may be sought.

Special Needs of Children with Multiple Handicaps

Most of the needs of Rachel, Edwin, Glenn, Diane, and even Debbie, who died at 7½ months, are similar to those of other, more fortunate, children: a loving family, a good home, a healthy environment, and expert and gentle medical care.

The coordination of care and planning is much harder for a child with several handicaps than for a child who has only one. Families may receive conflicting opinions from nurses, specialists, and the family doctor on such basic questions as the best time for surgery, the degree of the child's mental retardation, or the chances of the infant's living beyond the age of two. The family physician or pediatrician is often ideally placed to be the ombudsman in such situations, bringing together and synthesizing the various reports and presenting to the parents realistically what is known for sure and what is still a matter for ongoing study. The parents of a child with more than one handicap need expert advice on each defect and a coordinated, optimistic program to respond to the child's particular needs. Sometimes it is worth travelling a long distance, perhaps every one or two years, to a center where all the handicaps can be expertly reassessed and an updated plan developed and conveyed to the primary medical care group at home.

A planned approach, combining skill with realistic optimism and with empathy, one that confronts each problem as it arises yet never loses sight of the whole child and the child's future—this is the goal of good coordinated care. Families often display remarkable skills in learning from and teaching the health care team. When such a plan is achieved the child can be helped to reach his or her fullest potential.

Effective care for the child with multiple handicaps is costly and requires a considerable investment of time and energy from the family. Nevertheless, for most such children the gains that can be made in the quality of life are worth the cost.

Genetic Implications of Multiple Handicaps

When parents first realize that their child has more than one defect, they are overwhelmed by the new words they are constantly hearing and by their anxieties about how and when different problems can be treated. But soon questions arise about causes and implications for the rest of the family and for the future. These questions are even more pressing when a child has multiple handicaps than they are when a heart defect is the only problem.

Because so many syndromes involve the heart, it is impossible to go over the genetic implications of all of them. Here we can only summarize some general approaches; each child's individual problems and family history must be carefully assessed.

The presence of more than one defect does not necessarily mean the presence of a genetic syndrome. For example, an extra fifth finger is equally common in children with and without heart defects; a person born with an extra fifth finger and an atrial septal defect is no more likely to pass on a heart defect to a child than is someone who has an atrial defect alone. Parents of a child with multiple handicaps can use the checklist in chapter 3 to help them and their health team define the risk of a later baby's having a heart problem.

When a syndrome is present, it may be a Mendelian syndrome, meaning that a genetic cause has been identified, or it may be "sporadic," meaning that the syndrome does not run in the family and is unlikely to recur in the parents' next child or to be passed on to the offspring of the affected child. As more is learned about the human genome, it becomes evident that some syndromes are Mendelian at times and sporadic at other times; DiGeorge syndrome is an example. It is therefore vital that the genetic implications of the syndrome in a child be discussed with a geneticist or other expert.

In this chapter we have presented examples of children with chromosomal syndromes (Rachel and Edwin, both with Down syndrome [trisomy 21], and Debbie, with trisomy 13) and a family with a Mendelian syndrome (Glenn and his mother and brother, with Noonan-Ehmke syndrome). Diane had two severe problems, a central nervous system defect that caused loss of speech development and tetralogy with pulmonary atresia; she did not have a defined syndrome.

Down syndrome occurs in about 1 in 650 pregnancies. It is almost always due to an abnormality of chromosome division known as nondisjunction; the risk it will recur in the pregnancy is only about 1 percent. However, rarely—about 3 times in 100, Down syndrome is due to a translocation, that is, one parent is a carrier of a disturbance of chromosome 21. The recurrence risk in a subsequent pregnancy is then higher, more like 10 percent. The risk that Rachel herself will have an affected baby is high, around 33 percent.

Trisomy 13 is much rarer than Down syndrome; it is found in only one in seven thousand babies born alive. The risk that Debbie's parents will have another affected baby is only about 1 percent, but it would be advisable for Debbie's mother to have her chromosomes tested before she starts another pregnancy, because she is more likely than Rachel's mother to be carrying a translocation. Monitoring of any later pregnancy should include amniocentesis (early testing of the developing embryo's chromosomes). Infants like Debbie do not reach adulthood and do not have children.

Glenn's mother has Noonan-Ehmke syndrome herself, though in a mild form without any heart involvement. There is about one chance in two that any subsequent child of hers will have the syndrome. Glenn and his brother would have a similar risk of passing on the problem, although boys with the syndrome tend to be infertile. Glenn's sister, on the other hand, is unaffected and has no more chance of having a baby with the syndrome or with pulmonary stenosis when she grows up than does a friend or a neighbor.

Diane's two defects, involving heart and speech, seem to be sporadic. Even though tetralogy with pulmonary atresia is believed to be closely linked to abnormalities of the neural crest cells and developing nervous system, the risk that Diane's parents will have another child like Diane are less than 10 percent. Some children with speech and palate problems and tetralogy do have a rare syndrome known as Shprintzen syndrome, which is inherited similarly to Noonan-Ehmke, but Diane's speech defect is quite different. When Diane wants to have children of her own, she will have about a 10-percent risk of having a baby that has a heart problem, and she will need both cardiac reassessment and skilled obstetric advice at that time.

A large international project—the Human Genome Project—is under way to study exactly where each gene is situated on each of the forty-six chromosomes we all carry. The knowledge of the human genome is advancing faster than almost any other field of medicine, and this new information will help children with multiple handicaps and their families. As this knowledge accumulates, families can find encouragement in knowing how many parents have later had a normal child after having one with multiple handicaps. They can also be strengthened by the increasing attention and interest devoted to helping all handicapped children and adults. Support groups formed by families of such children have played a great part in bringing new and enlightened care to these children and in reminding teachers, politicians, and researchers of their special claim to our love and support.

Chapter 16

When Treatment Fails

As patients born with heart defects live longer—and begin to outlive the physicians caring for them—they rewrite what is written about natural history. As late as the late 1930s only a handful of people with tetralogy of Fallot reached middle age. Now there are hundreds of them, probably thousands, in all parts of the world. Many children born in the 1960s with transposition of the great arteries have lived to see their twenties; they have lived longer than almost anyone with transposition before them. A few children born with a hypoplastic left ventricle, one of the most severe heart defects, are now in their second decade of life.

Despite the great advances in management of childhood heart problems, death still occurs much more often in children with heart defects than in those born with normal hearts. Children who have additional defects outside the heart are more at risk. To take an extreme example, a baby with both trisomy 13 and a heart defect almost always (95 percent of the time) dies before the first birthday, regardless of any attempt to treat the heart itself. Almost one in five of the babies registered in the Baltimore-Washington Infant Study between 1981 and 1986 died before their first birthday. Someone who read the manuscript of this book exclaimed when she read this statement, "That figure seems very high, not consistent with the rest of the book. What explains this?" There are several reasons for this high figure, which we include not to alarm but to convey that although most heart defects are treatable, some are not. First, the cardiologists in the BWIS included in their study *all* of the infants they saw with heart defects, including those who had fatal problems outside the heart such as trisomy 13 or 18. (Many book chapters and booklets for parents omit these babies and concentrate on "isolated" heart defects. In some ways this is a good practice, because it keeps the emphasis entirely on the heart. We have not used it here, however, because it leaves out almost one in four of all children who are born with heart problems and also because in this book our focus is on the whole child.) Second, some of the mild congenital heart problems, such as atrial septal defects, may not be recognized in the first year of life, or the doctor may have heard a heart murmur in a healthy baby and not referred the baby for studies; these babies were not counted in the BWIS. Third, much of this book deals with childhood heart problems, that are completely benign, such as functional heart murmurs and mild arrhythmias. And fourth, it is true that most of the stories we have recounted here have been about successful treatment, or about children who did not need treatment at all. We have known for about thirty years that almost all deaths from heart defects occur in children under 1 year of age. In other words, the first year, and especially the first month of life, is the time of greatest risk, as the baby's heart and lungs adapt to the new life outside the womb. So the infants in the BWIS who reached their first birthday have a better than 95-percent chance of reaching adult life. They have passed without being aware of it through the "siege perilous" of infancy. As the BWIS continues into the 1990s, the percentage of babies who die young is decreasing each year, as more and more mild defects are recognized in early infancy and as every year more of the severe and the critical defects become treatable.

Amy S. was the first baby born to a young, healthy couple. Mrs. S. had had one previous miscarriage, but she felt well during this pregnancy and had no problems at delivery. Amy was full-term but weighed only 4.75 pounds. Immediately after birth she was very blue, and the level of oxygen in her blood did not improve when she was given oxygen. She was found to have dextrocardia. The radiologist noted that the liver shadow on the X-ray lay in the middle of the abdomen. Amy was started on prostaglandins and taken to a heart center, where she was diagnosed as having asplenia with an endocardial cushion defect, transposition, and pulmonary atre-

sia. She had a Blalock-Taussig shunt operation when she was 2 days old, and went home with an almost normal color.

Amy was put on a daily dose of penicillin, but she developed a number of ear infections and other infections nevertheless, and she grew poorly. Another shunt operation was performed when she was 3 months old. Open-heart repair was done when she was 3 years old. She died a few hours later.

Mrs. S. started a new pregnancy two years later, knowing that there was almost a one-in-four chance that any later baby would have a similar problem. The cardiologist had explained to her that when both the spleen and the heart have formed abnormally before birth, as they had in Amy, there is a complex looping defect of the heart, known as Ivemark syndrome. The heart problem often requires more than one operation; in addition, the syndrome is a Mendelian one, and the parents each carry a recessive gene and have almost one chance in four that the next baby will be similarly affected.

A fetal echocardiogram, done when Mrs. S. was twenty weeks pregnant, showed a large atrial septal defect with dextrocardia and heterotaxy (an abnormal arrangement of the liver and other organs in the abdomen). Mr. and Mrs. S. elected to end the pregnancy. The memory of Amy and all she had been through was too vivid to allow them to bring another child with a similar problem into the world.

Parents who have lost a child have written of their great sense of isolation. Even after Dr. Elizabeth Kübler-Ross wrote *On Death and Dying*, helping to breach the wall of silence the modern world has built around mortality, death in the young is hard to face. Many young adults have never personally known anyone, of any age, who has died. They may offer brief words of consolation to the grieving parents and then disappear. The parents feel abandoned in their grief. They feel that others' inability to talk about the loss and about the child is a denial of the meaning and significance of the parents' own lives. The health team can help alleviate some of these feelings by keeping in touch with the family, sometimes by attending the funeral service, by remaining available if new questions arise, and by being sure that a member of the family's support group is available.

When a child dies, more than one life is lost. The heart of the child stops beating and is still. With that death another life, the one the family shares with the child, also ceases. Even when a newborn infant dies, a whole world of dreams, imagination, and hope dies and is lost, for the parents have been planning and preparing since the pregnancy began or even long before. A mother who lost her 7-year-old son after his third operation for a complex heart defect wrote to us every Christmas of her "Little Drummer Boy." He was, like other beloved children, part of every legend and every fairy tale his parents knew. Even more distant relatives, grandparents and aunts and uncles, lose with the death of the child part of their own future, a relationship with the world, something gentle and intangible that can never be regained.

A friend of ours once wrote a one-act play called *Mark*, about a father and mother in the waiting area outside an operating room. Their 3-day-old son was having heart surgery. While they sat there, their hands clasped together, the father saw himself at an ice hockey rink, watching Mark, now 10 years old, leading his school team to victory. Mark's mother had her own dreams of Mark. These dreams—those they shared with each other, those they shared with the audience, and those they never told anyone—were part of the life that was Mark with his family. Only if Mark lived could that life go on. This drama is enacted in the real world every day; and, as in the play, we do not know the outcome.

The stress and grief may be even worse if the baby has already had several procedures and operations, only to die after weeks or even years. Then the parents lose that part of their past that was their dream of the future. If a child has been suffering, the parents know, despite their grief, that treatment had to be attempted. This sense of necessity, of having done all within their power to help, is a solace the family and health team can share together. If the child dies soon after birth or unexpectedly later, the family has had neither the time nor the opportunity to fully realize the danger and to prepare, and then acceptance may even be more difficult. If most of the child's brief life has been spent in intensive care, attached to monitors and intravenous tubing and equipment, the parents may feel haunted by the thought that they were not able to protect their child from pain, as their own parents had so lovingly protected them.

It is important for the health team to explain that heart pain is not a characteristic of childhood heart defects; children do not have angina, which adults experience when the heart muscle is not getting adequate blood flow through their blocked coronary arteries. The equipment, the intravenous tubing, and all the abnormal surroundings are not painful to the infant, even though the child is far from the gentle crib waiting at home. Some intensive care nurses have a special gift for recognizing that parents want to talk about some of their fears and feelings, and they help by showing they have the same concerns and are constantly alert to the baby's comfort, not only to the technology.

Death following a long chronic illness has other, more severe, effects. The parents may have removed themselves from many of their friends and activities in order to be with the child at the hospital or at home. When the child dies this new world is gone. One mother whose infant, Lisa, died after five months—all spent in intensive care—spoke of how much she missed the nurses and the sense of being part of a group that had fought so long and hard together. During those five months her own life had been in the intensive care unit; she was now like a weary veteran returning from the battle front, dreading normal life. She was helped in her reentry by a loving husband and by church friends who were not afraid to speak of loss and grief. She also joined a support group and began to work as a volunteer in a children's home. Her husband went with her to a few support group meetings but later chose to stay at home with their 6-year-old son, Carl, helping him with his homework while his wife went to the biweekly meetings. They were a close couple, and even though it was easier for her to talk about her feelings than it was for him, they never shut each other out. They both helped Carl recover from his own loss and his sense that he had been somehow abandoned while his baby sister was struggling for life.

When a child lives for many years with a heart defect and finally dies, from the defect itself or from further surgery, the parents experience additional shock and sorrow. The fact that so many hazards had been overcome, so many dangers outlived, gave them a sense that their child was somehow invulnerable. The parents fought hard for the child's life, battling not only the illness but sometimes methods of care they felt to be wrong; they may have sought out a number of health centers in search of help and encouragement. When death finally stops at the bed of their child, only a strong faith or personal philosophy combined with family love can slowly heal the parents.

The work of grieving is long and slow for loving parents. And grieving is exhausting. The sense of incompleteness, the loss of sleep, the constant thoughts of "if only," drain the energy of even young and strong parents. Their grief should never be belittled; they need acknowledgment and assistance. Sometimes reading about the similar suffering and exhaustion of others and talking it over with others helps to relieve the feeling of personal inadequacy that is a part of all intense mourning. Perhaps the only good to come from the terrible AIDS epidemic is an opening up of the subject of loss and grief so that others can share their experiences, and the acknowledgment that a young life lost casts so many shadows. Some communities have special support groups for parents who have lost an infant to sudden infant death syndrome or other causes. The group Lisa's parents attended, Big Hearts for Little Hearts, was organized by other parents of children with heart problems who had been treated at the same heart center at some time. Talking with others who had shared at least some of her experiences helped lift the sense of isolation Lisa's mother felt.

Parents rebuild their lives, and the work of grieving passes, although it never wholly ends.

Part IV

THE CHILD GROWS UP

Chapter 17

Living with a Heart Problem

Now that more children with heart defects are treated successfully in infancy, increasing numbers are reaching school age, adolescence, and adulthood. The overwhelming majority of those who reach
their first birthday are expected to have a normal life span. After a tu-
multuous start in life, they become part of the normal childhood population, with the same needs for family support, a good education, and
career planning. In past years the quality of life of a child born with a
heart defect was affected by the need for medication, staged operations,
and sometimes restrictions on activity, yet many such children, despite
some limitations during childhood, went on to fine careers in business
and the professions and raised families of their own.

More than six hundred thousand children and adolescents have repaired congenital heart defects. The parents of such children need to
learn how to help them live a full, active, and healthy life.

The Child in School

As more children have complete repair of heart defects in early infancy,
fewer enter kindergarten or first grade still needing major cardiac treatment. Changing patterns of child care, with more working mothers and
more day care, also mean that the transition from home to kindergarten
is a less traumatic event than in the past. Children are cared for in a
wide variety of settings. They spend more of their waking hours outside the home. It is important for parents to understand their child's

heart defect and be able to inform those caring for the child in school, day care, and elsewhere.

In spite of these changes, the parents of a child with any medical problem face questions and anxieties as the child enters a new environment. The time when a child starts school is an ideal time to clarify how well the heart is now functioning. This is true whether surgery has already been done or whether the issue is simply whether or not a heart murmur is innocent. It is also a time to determine whether future treatment is a possibility.

It is highly unlikely that any restrictions on the child's activity will be needed. By the time they enter school, most children who have had heart surgery in infancy can run and play actively with their peers. Rather, the question facing the family is usually what and how much to tell the school: Does the school need to know why Bobby has a scar on his chest, or how frequently Meredith needs to be seen by a cardiologist?

It is essential for the school to know that surgery has been performed, that it has been successful, and that full activity is possible and should be encouraged. This sharing and team approach avoids anxious speculation among the school staff and helps teachers to answer in an informed and helpful way any questions classmates may raise.

This postoperative group of children can be thought of as essentially healthy. With the help of the school they will blend in with their peers as easily as any other child.

For children who have not had surgery and will probably never need it, but who do have a loud heart murmur (most often as a consequence of a small ventricular septal defect), full participation in gym and sports is possible and is recommended. The school nurse should be made aware of the murmur and its cause; otherwise the nurse may hear it while checking the child after a fall or other incident at school and be alarmed.

A few children do still start school with a major heart problem. Perhaps it is a complex defect, one for which an operation may have been done but that still requires further corrective surgery. Perhaps it is a defect that results in blueness (cyanosis) of the skin and nail beds. Or a child may be smaller than other children of the same age and may need to be on medication to control signs of congestion and heart failure. There may be some disorder of the heart muscle that precludes the child's participation in sports. Or it may be that the child is normally well but nevertheless has repeated episodes of arrhythmia.

Krista had mild mitral valve prolapse and had attacks of atrial tachycardia about twice a year. She was an excellent swimmer and tennis player, and her attacks did not seem to be provoked by exercise. One day when she was 11 and sitting in history class, she began to feel her heart racing. The teacher noted that she was pale and sweating. Krista went to the nurse's office and tried all the maneuvers she knew to stop attacks: holding her breath, sipping ice water, even standing on her head, which had worked for her before. The school nurse measured Krista's blood pressure and heart rate and helped her try to come out of the attack, but nothing worked. The nurse called Krista's mother, who came and took Krista to the doctor's office. An electrocardiogram (EKG) confirmed that her heart rate was 240. The doctor told Krista he would give her an injection of adenosine. This had worked immediately once before, so Krista felt quite confident about having an injection, even though she cared little for needles. While the doctor was preparing the injection, Krista suddenly sat up, said, "I feel okay now," and felt her own pulse rate, now a normal eighty-two beats a minute. After repeating the EKG and letting her rest a while, the doctor let Krista go back to school.

Krista's story illustrates how the school, family, and physician—and Krista—all worked together as a team to help Krista miss as little school as possible.

The school health team approach

The school health team includes the school nurse, the physical education teacher, the classroom teacher(s), and the principal. The school nurse should be the first contact, as he or she will be called on to interpret the child's heart problem in the context of school experiences and activities. Each member of the team has an important role that is best defined in a group conference rather than in a series of one-on-one meetings. For difficult cases, or if the parents are unsure about how to discuss the problem, a heart center staff member, nurse, or physician can join in the conference.

The family and school need to share medical information about the child, relying on the following principles:

- All children must perceive themselves to be as much like their peers as possible.

- All children should do as much as they can. This is particularly true for children who are cyanotic; shortness of breath will limit how far or fast they can go. Restrictions imposed by the school are seldom needed.

- When restrictions of activity are necessary, alternative ways for the child to participate must be found: the child should have a special job or responsibility. In one school, a healthy twin played on the baseball team while his twin, who had an inoperable heart defect, was the coach's assistant. Each had a role, and each had the prestige that comes from being "on the team." The twin with the heart defect grew up and became a physician and lived to his late forties.

- For the child who has mild symptoms, the school, the family, and the cardiac treatment center need to maintain contact. A few well-planned phone calls often can lead to expeditious treatment and a reduction of stress for all concerned.

Collaboration between family and school

Collaboration between family and school is essential. The following examples indicate how well this collaboration can work.

A child with arrhythmia

Jimmy G. has Wolff-Parkinson-White syndrome and occasionally experiences episodes of rapid heart rate. Although these episodes are not dangerous for him, he does become pale and have to stop his activities until he can slow his heart rate. When the school nurse first heard about his problem she wanted to restrict his participation in gym and intramural sports. The heart center nurse clinician joined Jimmy's parents at a conference with school personnel and explained the nature of Jimmy's heart problem and the small risk of serious consequences. Now when Jimmy has an episode he reports to the nurse so that the school can keep track of the number of episodes. This information is helpful in adjusting his medication regimen.

It is important for the school to know if episodes of rapid heart rate or arrhythmia are likely to lead to other symptoms, and to know how urgent it is for the child to reach a treatment center when such episodes occur. It is most important to provide the school nurse with guidelines for a child's care. In most children of school age, an episode of tachycardia causes discomfort and sweating, but there is usually a safety margin of several hours. The parents will be able to take the child from the school sick bay to the heart center for help. Needless to say, it is much easier for the school nurse and teachers to be reassuring to the child if they know how long previous episodes have lasted and how they have been handled.

Many children become adept at returning their own rapid heart rates to normal through deep breathing, biofeedback techniques, or other maneuvers; needless to say, it is much easier for them if everyone around them is calm and well informed. Because arrhythmias are not uncommon, it is quite likely that one of the teachers in a large school will have experienced one or more episodes; such a teacher will be able to reassure the child and others. It is advisable to avoid inflammatory terms such as *heart attack*, for such terms convey alarming images of intensive care units or sudden death. Other terms, such as *paroxysmal tachycardia*, are too much of a mouthful; paraphrases such as "spells of rapid heart rate" can be substituted.

It is essential that the school become an integral part of the health team, helping to expedite treatment and minimize disruption of the child's years of growing and learning, when the child's self-esteem and sense of a normal body image are developing.

A child with a valvular heart problem

> Jake W. had heart surgery for aortic stenosis when he was 3 years old. He had done very well, and at 7 years old played as actively as his second-grade classmates. He had not been back to the heart center for more than two years; there had been a lot of family turmoil and resulting changes in insurance coverage in the meantime. His mother, who was now a single parent, planned to take him back for a checkup as soon as her insurance was in order again, perhaps in another six months.
>
> Jake was playing on the playground one day when he suddenly stopped playing, became very pale, and sat down. His teacher and the school nurse insisted that Mrs. W. take him that evening to his pediatrician. Although by that time Jake looked fine, the pediatrician was concerned that Jake's heart murmur had changed, and he arranged for Jake to be seen the next day by the cardiologist. The cardiologist found that the aortic valve repair was still satisfactory, but that Jake now had a severe obstruction in his left ventricle just below the valve.

Jake had surgery a few days later and recovered quickly. His classmates sent flowers and get-well cards, and his teacher arranged for lessons to be taken to his home for the short time he was to be out of school. The Children's Medical Services in the state where he lived was contacted, and they paid for the hospital expenses not covered by insurance. Jake's teacher arranged a welcome-back party when he returned to class.

The school played a vital role in helping Jake back to health, as schools have for many other children with heart problems. This story illustrates in addition how family turmoil may lead to difficulties in continued care. Mrs. W. had had a lot of things on her mind besides Jake's heart. She realized she had been told that he needed to see the cardiologist every year, but she did not fully understand why.

In the two years since his last visit to the cardiologist, Jake had changed, not only growing in height and weight but developing a more severe obstruction in his heart. His comfortable, stable, two-income family had changed as well: Mrs. W. was now a single mother with three children to care for, a very different constellation. Jake's insurance had also changed, although this should not have affected his care, because other help was available. The changes in Jake's family were more disruptive than those in most families, but no child grows in a vacuum and all families change somewhat with time. When family change is almost overwhelming, the school can be of great help in bringing the child's health back into focus.

A child who has cyanosis and is small for his age

John R. has a complex heart problem that has been helped by a series of heart operations, but his heart is not normal and he is small for his age, with a blue skin color and clubbing of the ends of his fingers. He also has a pronounced curvature of the spine.

In spite of his disability, John has a group of close friends. When the boys entered junior high, they decided to try out for the basketball team. John wanted to try out, but the school and John's parents were hcsitant, so his pediatric cardiologist went to a school conference and answered the questions of the school nurse and the physical education teacher. She told them that John would very likely become short of breath and be unable to keep up with the pace of the tryout, but that when he reached the limit of his exercise tolerance, he would stop and not harm himself. John tried out for the basketball team. He was disappointed that he was not among those chosen for the team, but then neither were any of his friends. They all tried, but none succeeded in making the basketball team. In John's eyes they are all the same. Now the five go to the basketball games together and root for their team.

Here the school played an important role in improving John's self-esteem by allowing him the room to grow that every adolescent needs.

A child with a family history of heart disease. Sometimes, however, the school may get only partial information and may react out of worry and concern.

Clara's father had a heart attack at the age of 35. With all the news in the media, her gym teacher was concerned that Clara might be at risk for an early heart attack. The teacher wanted Clara checked before she would allow her to participate in the physical education program at school. Clara's pediatrician reviewed her family history and physical examination and obtained a blood cholesterol level. All were normal, and he reported to the school that Clara should be allowed to participate in the physical education program.

Clara's pediatrician was the important member of the health team in this case; he provided the proper health information to the school and reinforced the need for education and facts. Although heart attacks occur frequently in some families, they almost never occur during the childhood years. Indeed, Clara's best defense against an early heart attack (**myocardial infarction**) is to establish lifelong habits of smoking avoidance, healthy diet, and cardiovascular exercise. Clara loves soccer, and she and her friends are members of the Smoke-free Class of 2000.

A child with an unrecognized heart problem. Rarely, an unrecognized heart problem in a child results in an event that can overwhelm the school.

Jim was an excellent student and a popular athlete. He had no known heart problem, and each year he passed his school physical examination for the sports teams. One day during basketball practice, however, he suddenly collapsed. His coach began cardiopulmonary resuscitation (CPR) immediately, but it was unsuccessful. As with all unexplained deaths, the county medical examiner or-

dered an autopsy. In the autopsy it was discovered that Jim's heart muscle was diffusely and severely thickened. He had a hypertrophic cardiomyopathy, and it is likely that he suffered a fatal arrhythmia.

Everyone in the school community was saddened and worried by the circumstances of Jim's death and wondered what they could have done differently. His parents agonized over why his heart abnormality had never been recognized. His coach worried that he had not performed CPR properly. His classmates and their parents worried that they, too, might die suddenly and without warning.

Each year about twelve students die suddenly in the United States during school athletic events. Although rare, these deaths receive extensive coverage in the newspapers and television and are widely discussed in the community. The rare heart defects that can put a child at risk include

- Hypertrophic cardiomyopathy, an unexplained massive thickening of the heart muscle
- Marfan syndrome, a congenital weakness of the supporting tissue of the body that can lead to ballooning of the aorta and to rupture
- Long QT syndrome, in which delayed electrical charges in the heart muscle can lead to ventricular tachycardia
- Single coronary artery, in which only one blood vessel supplies the heart muscle
- Other coronary artery abnormalities

In most cases there are no symptoms preceding these unexplained sudden deaths. But any of the following may be considered sufficient to alert the family and physician that a problem may exist:

- A family history of unexplained sudden death between the ages of 15 and 40. Heart attacks from coronary artery disease are infrequent in this age group, so sudden death is likely to be caused by another condition. Autopsy often shows severe heart muscle thickening.
- The physical appearance of Marfan syndrome. Children and adults with this syndrome are often said to resemble Abraham Lincoln: they are tall and have long arms and fingers, dislocated lenses in their eyes, and deformed chests.

- Unexplained frequent syncope (fainting) or atypical seizures. An electrocardiogram shows a characteristic lengthening of the QT interval. Other family members may also have an abnormal pattern.

Often after a tragic unexpected death like Jim's there is a call for screening of all students or all athletes. We must emphasize that such deaths are extremely rare. Further, to assess all children would be prohibitively expensive. For example, to screen all of the high school athletes in Rochester, New York, with a cardiologist's examination, EKG, and echocardiogram would require four pediatric cardiologists and six echo machines and would cost $2 million each year.

Explaining the Heart Problem to Family and Friends

One cause of agony for the parents of a sick infant is their inability to explain what is happening. Nearly every family has a Great Aunt Tilly or a Great Uncle Thad or some friend who is quick to jump to conclusions, swift to lay blame on a particular deed or person, and confident in their own broad medical background, gained from supermarket tabloids. Dealing with a sick child is difficult enough without the added burden of guilt brought on by uninformed people. The best defense is for a family to ask members of the heart center team all the questions that are lurking in their own minds. Parents often worry about asking silly or stupid questions. We want you to know that there is no such thing as a stupid question. Each question is real and therefore needs and deserves an answer, particularly in those first weeks and months after the initial diagnosis.

As the child gets older, parents face the question of how much to talk about the heart problem with family and friends and how to deal with follow-up visits to the cardiologist and the hospital. We return to the story of Jake W., the child with a valvular problem.

> *Jake had never really been told why he had a scar on his chest. When his classmates teased him about it he became upset. He was afraid to ask questions, for he had heard that his grandfather had had a chest operation for lung cancer, and he knew that a scar on the chest could mean something very bad.*
>
> *When Jake was suddenly readmitted to the hospital he felt a great deal of anger and fear. Fortunately, in this hospital there was an excellent program run jointly by the cardiac nurse specialist*

and the play therapist that used puppets and simple line drawings to explain to Jake the idea of a blockage in the heart and how such a blockage needed treating. Other ideas, such as the use of needles to give fluids for a short time after operations, were explained light-heartedly with the puppets. Of course, like all modern children of his age, Jake had seen medical programs on television, but this personal approach made everything seem more human and more real to him.

The health team and the family need to help the child understand his or her own heart. It is important not to overload the child with a lot of long words and elaborate explanations, but the child should know the exact name of the defect. The young child will accept quite cheerfully the idea that his or her heart has a problem that needs checking from time to time. By ten to twelve years, depending on the child's maturity, the responsibility for taking any medications should be primarily the child's. Taking responsibility for doing this is another part of the triangle of understanding (see Introduction). A properly presented explanation can empower a child, making him or her feel special. We know of one normal older sister who has asked when she, too, can have a scar showing how brave she was!

The Child Who Is Growing Slowly

Delayed growth caused by a heart problem is now much less frequent than it used to be. Most heart defects, as noted, can be corrected in infancy or early childhood, allowing normal growth of the rest of the body. But a child who is very small compared with others of the same age feels different and set apart. Parents and the school can help such children achieve a cheerful, outgoing disposition by helping them build a special niche for themselves, perhaps in music or art or schoolwork.

If both mental and physical growth are slow, there can be severe difficulties. Once it is clear that growth is slower than expected, it is useful for the child to have a thorough general checkup; it is possible that another problem, not the heart itself, is accounting for the delay in growth, and that this problem needs treatment.

We strongly encourage keeping a child with his or her peers in a mainstream classroom. Adaptive programs that allow a child to work to a different (lower) level of expectations often send a message that can reinforce a child's feeling of being different. If it is suggested to you that you place your child in an adaptive program, check with your heart center to see if this is for your child's benefit or for the school's.

Great Expectations

Every family has great expectations that the next generation will be better than its own. The newborn child is a focus of hope and joy for parents, grandparents, and the family constellation. If the newborn baby needs special care and heart surgery, the drama of these events may for a time cloud the family's expectations and make it hard to think of a hopeful future. Then when the child comes home, hopes and expectations rise again. Sometimes, indeed, expectations become inflated—the infant has survived so many perils that he or she must be very special, a superstar, a future prodigy. In this atmosphere it is extremely difficult to accept any setbacks, for example, signs that a baby or child is average or even a little slow. It is important for the sake of the child's and the family's future adjustment that the baby, and later the child, be treated as precious but as no more vulnerable or fragile than a healthy child.

The vulnerable-child label can follow a child long after successful repair of a heart defect. Because a child who was once ill is often perceived to be always defenseless, parents may constantly be anxious about threats from the environment and refuse to allow the child to take ordinary risks. One of the difficult aspects of parenting is to allow one's child to learn how to take reasonable risks. Denying such opportunity for growth can lead to a neurotic child and a neurotic family relationship. We encourage parents to discuss and face their fears and anxieties, perhaps with family counselling.

If the family and the health team have been too focused on the heart problem to have really seen the child as a whole, the start of school can be quite traumatic. If the school is the first to detect some learning problem and starts to talk of special tests or special classes, the family may feel resentful and may try to explain that the child's early surgery or other treatment is the cause. The health team should be monitoring the growth and development of a child so that if there is a learning lag it can be identified early and strategies can be developed to deal with it long before school starts.

The assessment of the child as a whole is crucial. The health team has an important role in helping the family develop a realistic idea of how the child will grow intellectually in the future; just as being born with a normal heart does not guarantee brilliance in school, neither does having a heart defect make it certain that a child will be a poor student. The primary physician is a key figure in helping the family fulfill the greatest of all expectations, seeing their infant grow into an active, lively, and treasured child with special gifts and talents.

Child to Teenager

Most children who are approaching adulthood today having had heart problems during childhood have already had their heart defects repaired. Others had defects too mild to require surgery. All of these children have become essentially normal young adults who have few, if any, residual problems. Some may have a scar on the chest and some a residual murmur over the heart, but all have taken part in normal school activities. An adolescent who has had childhood heart problems should know the name of the defect, whether there is a heart murmur, and whether any abnormality appears on an electrocardiogram. This knowledge will prevent unnecessary anxiety if a new physician is encountered, as happens so frequently in today's mobile society. Students going away to college or young adults starting out in a new environment should carry with them a note summarizing the relevant details of their last evaluation, advice on how frequently cardiac reevaluation is necessary and whether or not BE prophylaxis should be given, and the name of a physician or cardiologist who can be contacted if necessary.

Occasionally a teenager with a small ventricular septal defect will show symptoms in early adult life, and surgical repair of the defect may then be recommended. Or, infrequently, a child with a mitral valve prolapse will develop more mitral insufficiency and need valve repair. But for the most part, children with such problems continue to do very well into adult life; cardiac follow-up will usually be needed at two- to five-year intervals, the length of the interval varying with the nature of the problem.

Some teenagers and young adults have heart problems that do require continued cardiac care and supervision. For some who have had surgery an additional problem remains, such as a leaking heart valve or a septal defect. Others have heart problems that tend to progress in severity, for example, everyone who has aortic valve disease, even if surgery has already been done. Such children are at some risk that the problem will become more severe over time. Symptoms themselves are not a reliable indicator of whether or not a valve is functioning well. Any child who has an artificial valve or any enlargement of the heart or who is still blue (cyanotic) needs continued follow-up, preferably at a center already well informed about the specific problem. Any teenager who is taking anticoagulant (blood-thinning) medications or who has repeated abnormalities of heart rhythm also needs careful and consistent advice.

It is particularly important that the teenager who has a heart problem be comfortable with the cardiac health team and know that members of the team are readily available by telephone.

Chronic illness in adolescence

Another group, few in number but needing a great deal of care, have heart defects for which no standard surgical repair is available. Some of these teenagers may be eligible for a future heart or heart-lung transplantation. Others will have multiple medical complications, some directly related to the heart and some to other parts of the body. In such cases, as in all cases of adolescents with chronic illness, a special kind of health team approach is needed.

Some physicians are ill at ease with a teenager whose severe health problem is superimposed on the normal mood swings and rebelliousness of adolescence. Other physicians feel a sense of personal failure because there is no operation available that will cure the defect; unconsciously and unfortunately, these physicians may transmit an atmosphere of gloom. Ideally, the primary-care physician will be one who has special skill with adolescents and who can collaborate with the cardiac team on a long-term course, assuming that such a course is realistic. The emphasis needs to be on the positive aspects of what can be done and on obtaining the best quality of life in the years available. The family of a young person with no clear available cure is already facing many anxieties, and they need to be helped to permit their child to mature and to make decisions. Such teenagers may not say exactly what their frustrations are, but they are well aware of the difference between their own activity level and that of their schoolmates. The family and the health team need to develop a close, cheerful, and friendly relationship with such teenagers, respecting their privacy yet remaining open to discussing troublesome or even minor symptoms.

Most of the time, although those who are chronically ill may have a shortened life expectancy, the actual duration of life cannot be predicted. It is therefore of great importance to plan for the long term, encouraging academic development and activities to maintain muscle tone and strength and encouraging as normal a social life as possible. Indeed, the principles of helping a teenager with a chronic heart problem and a deteriorating heart are exactly those so extensively written about for helping victims of AIDS or childhood malignancy. The principal theme is that a life, even if short, can be intense, productive, and happy, and an inspiration to others. This theme has been movingly expressed in books written by parents of children dying in their teens of cancer, including John Gunther's *Death Be Not Proud*.

The teenage years and entrance to adulthood are affected by the severity of the child's heart problem. Thus, except for needing a cardiac checkup every few years, the teenager with a trivial defect or one who has had successful surgery has little more difficulty than others of his age, whereas those with more severe heart defects may have delayed growth, may be limited in sports or in keeping up with their peers, and may experience difficulty in school from side effects of medications or from the necessity of frequent hospital visits and surgery.

All of these adolescents, whatever the expectations for resolution of their heart problem, face the same needs as their friends. They need a good quality of life with good psychosocial adjustment. Later, as young adults, they need to establish an independent life and get a job. Many will start a new family constellation and a new generation. These are daunting challenges for everyone, with or without a heart problem.

The quality of life in the teenage years is overwhelmingly affected by the patterns of schooling and family cohesiveness in the early years of childhood. A child who attended school regularly and made acceptable grades will have a sense of achievement and self-worth. Absenteeism and school problems, on the other hand, will lead to a downward spiral that is somewhat worse for an adolescent with a heart problem than for one with a normal heart; teachers and family both will then wonder how much the heart problem can be blamed. Because the teenage years are difficult at best, it is essential to establish early in life whether any school absences can reasonably be expected for cardiac reasons. This is an important step for all of these children, but particularly for a child who has some learning disability in addition to a heart defect, for in the teenage years it is harder to go to school if one is slower than average.

The family of a child with a heart problem should be constantly vigilant and encouraging, helping the child in every way possible to become a full participant in school and home life. Those teenagers with heart problems who enjoy the best quality of life have parents who show great expectations but do not push their child beyond his or her potential.

Psychosocial adjustment

In addition to the usual tumults of adolescence, teenagers with heart problems may have unresolved questions about body image, about their changing relationships with their families, and about whether their heart problems will prevent them from becoming normal adults. Most such adolescents deal in a matter-of-fact way with the scars from surgery. Only in a minority is the scar a focus of their own and parental worries, and in such cases plastic surgery may be helpful. If there are other visible signs of an underlying heart problem, such as a blue color to the skin or clubbing of the fingers, these problems can be accepted as challenges to be overcome or ignored. But some adolescents may need counselling, ideally by an adolescent counselor who has knowledge and experience with teenagers who have chronic physical handicaps.

One of the hardest tasks for all adolescents is to adjust to their new role in the family, and to resolve the conflicts that naturally arise between dependence and independence. Most children with heart problems that are corrected in infancy have no unusual difficulty in achieving normal independence as they mature. However, adolescents who have chronic illness of any kind have a less easy time, because they will continue to be somewhat dependent on their families for hospital visits, purchasing medications, and even for personal care. In the most successful families with a chronically ill child, the teenager accepts responsibility for taking medications and scheduling appointments. Some studies have shown that excessively dependent chronically ill teenagers risk developing a difficult family relationship, one in which the parents gradually become withdrawn and fail to provide needed emotional support. When a chronically ill teenager seems in danger of too great a dependency, family counselling may help.

A successful adult life will involve employment and the establishment of enduring relationships outside the family unit. In past years employers and insurance companies looked askance at individuals with heart problems, but now few jobs are closed to a young man or woman who has had successful heart surgery or who has a minor heart defect. The Natural History Study II found that children with ventricular septal defects, with aortic stenosis, and pulmonic stenosis, who were followed for an average of twenty-two years, had employment histories as adults that were similar to those of other members of their families. Almost 80 percent were either in college or fully employed at the time of the follow-up study. Similarly encouraging reports are available about adults who had prior surgery for tetralogy of Fallot and other severe heart problems.

For the rare individual with a chronic heart problem for whom full-time employment is impossible, income from Social Security Disability allowances will help greatly in establishing independence. It is extremely difficult for such people to find good supplementary part-time work. Some can work in sheltered workshops, but because most of the other workers there are mentally retarded, such workshops will not provide the kind of collegial companionship the child with a chronic heart problem has had during the school years. Making productive use of the skills of the chronically ill is an issue that has not yet been adequately dealt with.

The teenager with a heart problem may have more than the usual anxiety about sexual relationships. Still, except in a few syndromes, the fertility and sexual performance of people with heart defects are quite normal. And although in the past marriage and pregnancy often occurred later for individuals born with heart problems than for their classmates, this difference will probably disappear in the future years, because the age for marriage and childbearing in the general population is rising and the age at which heart defects are repaired is declining.

For young women with heart problems the best method for contraception was once a topic of considerable concern, but it is now clear that the overwhelming majority of such women have no special risks in this respect; they can use the same methods available to others. Women who have artificial heart valves, who have enlarged hearts, or who remain blue or cyanotic do have special problems; for example, oral contraceptives are not advisable. Teenagers who fall into these categories need skilled and well-informed gynecologic consultation. In most stable relationships a satisfactory method of contraception involving both partners can be found; for young women in unstable relationships, or those with multiple defects, tubal ligation may be an option.

Social Problems

Almost all children born today with heart defects can look forward to a long and healthy life. Major problems remain for children with complex defects, including those with hypoplastic left or right ventricles,

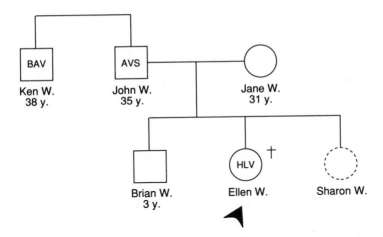

17.1. The W. Family. In this diagram males are shown by *squares*, females by *circles*, and the *arrow* indicates the original, or index, patient (the person first seen by the physician). Sharon W., who had no heart defect, was born two years after Ellen's death. *Key: BAV* = bicuspid aortic valve; *AVS* = aortic valve stenosis; *HLV* = hypoplastic left ventricle.

and for children with multiple defects that include the heart (see chapter 15).

Children with heart defects may still have difficulty in obtaining insurance coverage. Unfortunately, because the excellence of the outlook for children with mild defects is not as widely known as it should be, even children whose defects cause no physical problems may have such difficulties.

The problems of a child born with a heart defect thus are not limited to the defect. They include

- The heart defect itself
- Society's reaction to the defect
- Ethical issues arising from a severe defect or multiple handicaps
- Genetic and family implications

These problems interact with each other in a multitude of different ways, as illustrated by the W. family, whose family tree is shown in figure 17.1 and whose story is told below.

The W. family included three members with left-heart flow defects, all leading to quite different problems. Kenneth W. is now 38 years old. He has a bicuspid aortic valve that has never given him any trouble. He played games in school, was a good student, and now is an active member of a law firm; he has group insurance. His younger brother, John W., has mild aortic valve stenosis, but he also has been free of heart symptoms. He has his own business and has had enormous difficulty in obtaining life insurance; the health insurance premiums quoted to him are too high for his income. His child, Ellen, who had a hypoplastic left ventricle, has insurance because of her mother, Jane W.'s job with a bank that has extensive group coverage.

Ellen's heart defect was discovered when she was 3 days old, just as she was about to leave the hospital. She suddenly became pale and mottled, having previously seemed vigorous. Tests showed that she had a tiny left ventricle. She was started on prostaglandin treatment and her color improved. Physicians and nurses reviewed with the family the diagnosis and possible treatment plans. The parents were confronted with a terrible dilemma—should they embark on a long and difficult course for treatment that could require going to another city for a long hospital stay? Neither heart transplantation nor the Norwood operation was available locally. While they were pondering what to do, with much help from their family, their friends, and their church group, they learned that Ellen did not have normal chromosomes. She had Turner syndrome (XO chromosomes, not XX as in a normal girl). Although this syndrome was not life-threatening, it did mean that she did not have normal ovaries and could never have a child. Later in childhood she would need hormone medications to help her grow to average height. The family had to think not only of how they and Ellen would deal with Ellen's future, but of how her treatments and the travel back and forth for her cardiac care would affect little Brian, her 3-year-old brother, who would have to be left with others. They decided to go ahead with surgery and went to the heart center 200 miles away. Ellen did well after the Norwood operation. She returned home a month later but then developed a serious virus infection and died at the age of 5 months.

A few months after her death her parents sought advice about future children. They were anxious to have another child, even after they learned that the risk of that child's having a heart defect was between 10 and 20 percent. They followed the advice given

*them about a next pregnancy and fortunately had a healthy little
girl two years after Ellen's death.*

This story illustrates how the severity of the heart defect influences
family decisions. For Kenneth W. and his brother, problems so far have
mainly involved battles over insurance premiums and the minor nuisance of taking BE prophylaxis. The question of insurability is much
less of a problem than it once was. The American Heart Association has
held meetings over the years with large insurance companies to present
the newest information on long-term outcomes of particular defects.
Nevertheless, insurance problems still exist, as evidenced by an insurance company's recent letter to a cardiologist about a healthy 4-year-old
boy who has a tiny ventricular septal defect. The boy was offered insurance on his father's policy, but any problems related to his heart were
excluded. The letter reads:

> Dear Doctor,
>   Thank you for your further information about Joseph X.
> We regret we cannot offer him full coverage, since complica-
> tions may be caused by his heart defect.
>   Yours sincerely,

The principal problems caused by mild heart defects are societal,
involving insurance, school acceptance, and similar issues. Occasionally, societal and family problems overlap, as revealed in a letter of
application for Social Security Disability benefits for a 10-year-old girl
who has a heart murmur but in whom no abnormality of any kind is
apparent on a chest X-ray, electrocardiogram, or echocardiogram:

> Sheena has a murmur over her heart, and her family is afraid to
> let her play, in case she is hit over the heart.

We do not know how well the health team that has seen Sheena
tried to explain to the family that her innocent heart murmur did not
mean disease (see chapter 9). Did they perhaps hurry Sheena through
the system, subjecting her to a barrage of electrocardiograms, echo-
Dopplers, and other high-tech procedures that the family had seen associated on television with life-and-death illness, and then spend only
two minutes telling the family, "She's fine; nothing to worry about. Just
a heart murmur"? Perhaps they spent a lot of time talking to the family;
they may have given Sheena's mother the American Heart Association

booklet and been convinced that everything was clear. However conscientious the health team was, communication and understanding were not achieved.

When the heart defect is severe and life-threatening, as in the stories in this chapter, ethical and practical questions may overwhelm the family. How much should they sacrifice, in time, money, and emotion, to save an infant who will never have a normal heart? How much importance should be given to future psychosocial questions, such as a child's restricted activity, possible lack of acceptance from friends, and later problems including employment, insurance, and possibly an inability to establish a family? If Ellen's parents accept the fact that while they are with Ellen in a hospital miles away they cannot be with her 3-year-old brother, how much should they ask little Brian to sacrifice now? Such dilemmas cannot be resolved simply. Cardiologists and others on the health care team are deeply divided over the answers. If, for example, Ellen's problem had been diagnosed before birth after a fetal echocardiogram, would the parents have chosen to end the pregnancy? How can parents be helped to reach such a decision, and who can best help them? Suppose Ellen had had a different chromosomal problem, one associated with mental retardation; how certain need the health team be of the severity of the retardation and the impaired quality of the child's life before they advise the parents that intervention is not in the family's best interest?

None of these issues is unique to the child with a heart defect. But each family faces its own unique problems. In the future, as diagnosis and surgical techniques reach an even higher level of achievement, the nature and type of ethical issues involved will change. As knowledge about the successful outcome for most heart defects becomes more widespread, societal questions about insurance and restriction of a child's activity will decrease, but as it becomes possible to save more and more children with complex conditions, other questions about quality of life may take their place.

The increasing interest shown by society as a whole in helping handicapped children lead a full life has been a great boost to many such children and their families. But a special form of bonding is needed between the family and the health team, and between these adults and the child, when the child has a complex problem. The combination of good humor, patience, and realistic optimism shown by many such children inspires the other members of the triangle of understanding. In the future more intensive outreach programs will be available to help children receive more and more of their needed treatments at home. Infants and children who need prolonged and complex treatments constitute fewer than one-third of all those with heart problems who are admitted to a hospital for care, but they are an important minority and are in need of continuing research, innovations in methods of care, and understanding for them and their courageous families.

The Next Generation: Having Children of Their Own

The subject of their own children's children is a topic that occurs to all parents as soon as their own child is born, but parents whose child has a heart problem will face it with special concern. "Can she have children?" "Will her children be normal?" Such questions are frequently asked soon after an original diagnosis of a heart defect is made.

The answer is that almost all young people who were born with heart defects are capable of having children. Only a very few will have a disorder such as Noonan-Ehmke syndrome (see chapter 15), which is associated with infertility in boys, or Turner syndrome, which is associated with infertility in girls. So the ability to have children, fortunately, exists, and we have felt it important, as part of the heart center evaluation for a child around ten to twelve years of age, to remind the family of this ability. Frank discussions of the responsibilities of childbearing, and of the need for young people to postpone these responsibilities until their own home can be established, are important in all families and school settings, but possibly even more so for young adults with heart defects. A poorly educated young woman with a heart defect will find it hard to become a good mother. The search for love and acceptance may push her to an early teenage pregnancy. To a teenager with a heart problem, particularly if she has family difficulties or a learning disability, a baby may well seem a loving uncritical gift in a harsh and troublesome world. Helping her to realize that she can be a better mother, probably an excellent mother, if she waits is an important way to help her become a healthy adult.

Pregnancy can be dangerous to women who have certain types of heart defects, including high pressure in the lungs (Eisenmenger syndrome) or severe heart muscle disease (cardiomyopathy). In addition, the presence of an artificial heart valve will require significant precautions to maintain the health of both mother and infant. But with these few exceptions, most young women with heart problems will have no added difficulties during pregnancy or delivery.

Will the child be normal?

Early studies of children born to a parent who has had heart problems were very reassuring: a young adult born with a heart problem had only about a 5-percent chance of bearing a child with a similar defect. This was true whether the new parent was the father or the mother, provided that the other parent had a normal heart and that neither family had other members with heart problems. However, two more recent studies have indicated a higher risk of a heart defect in the next generation, closer to 14 percent. Why such a discrepancy exists is still uncertain. The optimists among researchers think that the new studies are wrong, that they may have included, by chance, too many "high-risk" families; the pessimists think the early studies were not thorough enough. Whom should one believe, and what is the best advice?

First, no matter which studies are correct, the baby of a parent who has had a heart problem has at least an 80-percent chance of having a normal heart. Second, most heart defects are mild and do not need surgery. Third, in about two of three cases a defect in the child is concordant with (closely similar to) that in the parent. Thus if a young man or woman with a small ventricular septal defect, for example, has a baby, there is a high probability that if the baby also has a defect, it will be mild and will not require surgery.

The time when the couple decides to start a new family is a good time for a detailed cardiac checkup. Both partners can then review together the exact nature of the heart problem. In a few complicated situations an additional consultation with a geneticist is important. If both parents have a defect the risk is more than doubled; fortunately, this situation is surprisingly unusual, and it is quite complicated to discuss because the risk depends on the genetics of the defect in each. In such cases the prospective parents should consult their doctors. It is helpful also to choose an obstetrician who has experience with women with heart murmurs or other such health problems. These obstetricians are sometimes called high-risk obstetricians, though this is an unfortunate term: they are a special group who are happy to work with cardiologists and other physicians to ensure the best possible outcome for mother and baby. Early registration for prenatal care and avoidance of any risk factors likely to damage the developing heart are also important. A fetal echocardiogram at sixteen to twenty weeks, if done in a center with special expertise in looking at the heart, can also be helpful and reassuring to the prospective parents.

It should be immensely reassuring to the young couple to know that the great majority of children born with heart defects can now reach adulthood and experience for themselves the joys of becoming the parents of normal children.

The Pioneer Patient

Pioneer physicians and surgeons cannot exist without pioneer patients. If a treatment is new and exciting to the medical world, it is by necessity even newer, more exciting, and more perilous to the child and the family. The pioneer patients of the 1940s and 1950s who first underwent the "blue baby operation" are now beyond the middle of their lives, themselves have children now out in the world.

Mary W. first came to Baltimore as a 5-year-old child. She had been blue, or cyanotic, from birth and had had some severe spells of blueness and shortness of breath when she was between 6 and 18 months old. She could walk only about one block before squatting down on her haunches to rest. In all other ways she was a lively, alert little girl. Her parents, who lived in Pennsylvania, had read of the new "blue baby" operation and came to see if it would help Mary. The year was 1947.

Dr. Helen Taussig examined Mary and found she had tetralogy of Fallot and had a good chance of being helped by surgery. Dr. Blalock performed the Blalock-Taussig shunt operation (first performed in 1944). Mary's color improved and she went to school and acted like a normal child, returning every year or two for checkups. She always had a slightly blue tinge to her skin, but was very active.

In 1960 Mary became blue again, having to some extent outgrown her previous operation. Open-heart repair of tetralogy had only been done for five years, and the operation still carried a risk of greater than 20 percent. Mary pioneered again, and again had an excellent course after operation. Her color was now normal and the function of her heart excellent.

She married and had four healthy children and one miscarriage. In 1984 her father, who had always been healthy, became unable to garden because he was so short of breath. Mary was sure he had a heart problem and should get treatment. He was not easy to persuade, being a stoical man of Scots-American extrac-

tion. Mary, her husband, and her mother escorted him to Baltimore to see a cardiologist. To everyone's surprise and delight, Mr. M. was short of breath from anemia due to a bleeding gastric ulcer. His heart was fine. He did well, and talked with pride of Mary, his son-in-law, and his grandchildren.

Mary came with her family to the memorial service held for Dr. Taussig in 1986 in Baltimore and spoke movingly of her early memories of and her later friendship with someone who had been to her more than a physician. There were some fine speeches on that occasion, but Mary alone could speak for the pioneers.

It is not given to every pioneer to do so well or to be able to reward her parents and her physician so remarkably. But every pioneer has something to teach us. We have all learned from Elias G., who came with his parents from Poland to escape the Holocaust and who works every day in an office despite intense cyanosis; from Louise M., who faced most of the complications we have discussed, and many we have not, with gallantry and sardonic humor; and from many, many others who have forged the way when the outcome was hard to see. Rather than generalizing about them, we append here some excerpts from a recent videotaped interview by one of us (EBC) with Carol S., a medical social worker with a complex congenital heart defect. She has unique insight into the dynamics of interaction among patients, family, school, and the health care team.

Talking about her visits to the pediatric cardiologist, Carol said:

> It was always very frightening—I never felt very sick or different except when I went to Children's. It reminded me every time that they didn't have a lot of answers. The older I got, the more I resented going.

Talking about people's response to her, she recalled:

> For years strangers would walk up to me and say, "Do you know your lips are purple?" As if I didn't know that—it was extremely rude. I don't know why people do that, but I had it [those comments] for years, especially from school teachers.... I think as a little kid I didn't realize, but when I was older I would get sarcastic.

Carol described her teenage years this way:

When I was a teenager school became harder and harder. I wasn't sick then in terms of being in and out of the hospital. I was tired all the time and it was very hard for me to go to school for a whole week. My grades were fine, I was keeping up on everything...it was just really frustrating. It took me years to realize that I was tired...I always felt my friends and teachers thought I was faking.... If you are not in a wheelchair or have a guide dog, [people consider that] you are not really physically handicapped. This is very hard for people to understand. I wish it had been different, but I left school in tenth grade. I didn't quit because I didn't want to learn. I quit because it was just frustrating.

She had difficulty communicating with physicians:

There was never any discussion—they would say, "You are doing fine," that's it. No one wanted to make any plans for me or to tell me what I was facing in the future. I went to my cardiologist, asked him these questions, and he never got back to me. He never called me back.

Carol's message to all health caregivers is this:

Patients like me have a chronic illness.... Give me credit for understanding it and for having lived with it and knowing something. This [the cardiac defect] is my whole life.... Doctors want to take over all the controls. They want to have everything. When things don't go right,...it is very easy for them to say, "You are not trying hard enough." I want someone I can really trust, kid around with and really know something about and feel that he is one of the more important people in my life. With a chronic illness, you have to have that.

As patients grow and thrive and enter their adult years, we physicians often lose sight of the complexity of their lives. We continue to think of them as the infant with a "heart defect," not as an integrated member of society—a husband, wife, friend, parent, colleague—whose life is complicated by and often dominated by the burden of a congenital **cardiovascular** defect. Their reactions to caregivers, teachers, family, and friends include anger, frustration, and endurance. We believe one of our challenges is to *accompany* our patients in their lives, allowing them to make their own choices. This is their right.

Chapter 18

Living with
a Healthy Heart

The healthy heart of a child is one of life's great wonders. Watching the heartbeat of a healthy newborn baby or observing the overwhelming energy of a 10-year-old, we realize the marvels of the normal circulation before age or atherosclerosis have touched it. How can we help a child keep the healthy heart of youth? How can we help a child who has had a heart defect maintain his or her new-found health?

Some persons who are interested in the aging process have calculated the number of heartbeats "programmed" from before birth until natural death at 85 years or so to be 2.7 billion! We are all interested in keeping those billions of heartbeats healthy.

There is great popular interest in heart health. This is partly because heart attacks often afflict people in their most productive years, partly because we know that heart disease and stroke are great killers and cause much illness in the Western world, and partly because of the publicity about the success of recent heart surgery. The success of non-surgical treatments such as balloon dilation of the coronary arteries (coronary **angioplasty**) has also been much publicized. But perhaps the greatest interest comes from the knowledge that much heart disease can be *prevented* by healthy living; indeed, it is impossible to read a popular magazine or watch television without being reminded of the benefits of exercise, the hazards of **obesity**, the dangers of a diet high in saturated fats and cholesterol, and the dangers of smoking cigarettes.

We assume that our readers are familiar with these general topics.

Our focus is how to help a child keep that wonderful gift, a healthy heart, and to help a child who was born with a heart defect maintain a heart that has been restored to a near-normal state. Maintaining a newly healthy heart is a project scarcely imaginable a few short years ago, when few children with heart defects reached adulthood.

This goal is equally important for all members of the family. It is never too early or too late to begin a program for a healthy heart.

We start by accepting that some slowing of the heart rate, especially in the maximum response to exercise, and some loss of elasticity of the walls of the arteries are inseparable from the aging process. But in most of us, these changes occur to a greater degree than is necessary. How can we maintain a healthy heart as we age? What increases the risk of heart disease in future years? And what can we do to prevent heart disease?

Prevention of certain disorders (for example, atherosclerosis, hypertension, and diseases of the heart muscle) is irrevocably linked to the maintenance of cardiovascular health. Analogies between the heart and the automobile are generally inappropriate, but the maintenance of both does involve care and vigilance. A healthy, "tuned-up" heart is a source of joy and prevents future trouble. Starting early is crucial.

Prevention of Atherosclerosis

Atherosclerosis is a complex process. In the newborn infant the coronary arteries have a completely smooth inner lining that allows blood to flow freely to every area of the heart. As the years pass, irregular patches, or *plaques*, appear in the lining of arterial walls. Such plaques recognized in the aortas and large arteries of young men in their early twenties who died in the Korean War provided an early clue that atherosclerosis was not simply a disease of old age, but began in youth. The word *atherosclerosis* comes from the Greek *a there* (mushy, like gruel) and *skleros* (hard). It reminds us that at first the arteries contain small soft deposits of fat, chiefly cholesterol; later these deposits become larger and begin to accumulate fibrous material that is similar to scar tissue, causing the arteries to harden and thereby to lose the elasticity of youth. The arterial wall also becomes thicker.

Plaques begin to appear in the coronary arteries—usually in the left coronary artery first—when a person is about 15 years of age. By the third and fourth decade of life these plaques become widespread throughout the coronary tree (figure 18.1). If a clot forms over one of

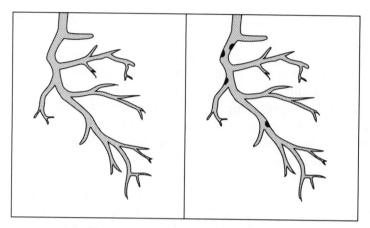

18.1. Coronary Atherosclerosis. *Left,* Healthy left coronary artery without plaques; *right,* plaques blocking branch of left coronary artery.

these plaques, leading to a **coronary thrombosis** or vessel blockage, the heart muscle supplied by the blocked artery is deprived of necessary blood and a heart attack occurs.

More often there is not a sudden blockage, but a gradual reduction in blood flow through one or both coronary arteries. The arteries silt up, rather like a muddy river or a contaminated water pipe. The patient, most often a previously healthy middle-aged man, can no longer undertake his regular activities without chest discomfort or pain. His now narrowed coronary arteries do not allow sufficient blood flow during exercise. He is diagnosed as having angina pectoris (chest pain due to coronary insufficiency).

Atherosclerosis in the arteries to the brain can lead to *stroke.* A single large clot can result in a major stroke, with paralysis of one side of the body; progressive silting up of the brain arteries can cause a series of "little strokes" and steady deterioration of brain function, somewhat similar to Alzheimer's disease. When atherosclerosis attacks the leg arteries, in peripheral **vascular** disease, severe leg pain may result.

Most atherosclerosis is preventable. A statement like this irritates some people. "Oh, you think if we all lived on vegetables and fish oil we'd live to be 110 years old. I'd rather enjoy life while I have it." Or, "My neighbor has always jogged and is thin and healthy looking, but he had a massive heart attack a month ago. He's only 38 years old. Jogging and keeping thin hasn't done much for him."

It is unfortunately true that some families have a high risk of heart attacks, usually because of genetic cholesterol problems. These families need special follow-up and medication. Jogging and diet alone won't be enough. Dr. Peter Kwiterovich's book *Beyond Cholesterol* (Johns Hopkins, 1989) explains how genetic problems may lead to familial hypercholesterolemia. But the overwhelming majority of families can maintain heart health for themselves and their children without strenuous dieting or medications.

In the 1960s, from an important study of everyone who lived in Framingham, Massachusetts, scientists gradually learned that certain factors of lifestyle, diet, and **heredity** increased the risk of heart attack. This was a large epidemiologic study of a defined population of people, comparing adults who had some history of atherosclerosis or heart attacks with those who had none. The study began in 1949; by the 1960s the findings about risk factors were beginning to be published. In addition to factors that are not controllable—age, male gender, family history of early heart attack—the researchers found other risk factors that *can* be controlled, especially smoking, high blood levels of cholesterol, and hypertension (high blood pressure). Many subsequent studies have confirmed these risk factors in other populations in the United States and in other countries as well. Lack of exercise, obesity, diabetes, and low levels of **high-density lipoprotein** (HDL, sometimes called alpha-cholesterol, or "good cholesterol") were also found to add to the risk of atherosclerosis. A new field of medicine, preventive cardiology, was developed to deal with reducing such risk factors.

High blood pressure may make atherosclerosis worse, probably by increasing the stress and strain on the coronary artery walls, and it can also lead to kidney disease or to stroke. Unless there is a strong family predisposition to high blood pressure, it can be avoided in childhood by moderating salt intake and engaging in regular exercise. Medication for hypertension is rarely needed in children or adolescents.

The Family's Role in Keeping the Child's Heart Healthy

It was some time after the Framingham study before the concept of risk factors became generally accepted. It was even longer before the acceptance of another idea, the theme of this chapter and an idea that now seems so very obvious: Childhood is the best time to start keeping a healthy heart, because the heart is usually still healthy in childhood.

We consider in this chapter especially the risk factors of smoking and diet.

Cigarette smoking

Smoking is the largest and most easily controlled risk factor for coronary and atherosclerotic heart disease. Smoking has several effects on the heart. A smoker's first puff in the morning makes the heart race and the fingers tingle, a direct consequence of nicotine and catecholamines, powerful natural stimulating chemicals that speed the heart and constrict the blood vessels in the hands and feet and also the coronary arteries, reducing blood flow to the heart muscle itself. Constant exposure to the toxic chemicals in cigarette smoke damages the lungs and reduces the blood's ability to carry oxygen to the body and particularly to the heart muscle. In some people with already narrowed coronary arteries, the resulting spasm can produce angina or even trigger a heart attack. Those who say "I'll quit when I have my first symptom" should remember that the first sign in about 50 percent of people who die from heart disease is SUDDEN DEATH from an irregular heartbeat.

Young people begin to smoke because they see their parents or other role models smoking and because they see advertisements that link smoking to "cool" or sophisticated adult behavior. The tobacco industry spends millions of dollars to encourage the consumption of cigarettes. There is an expanding market for cigarettes now among teenage girls, who are lured by ads that show women smoking in exotic settings. Many teenagers are encouraged to smoke by peer pressure from their friends. Those who smoke are likely to have friends who smoke.

> *Christabell's parents, Tom and Jane, have smoked since their late teens. Christabell is in third grade and has learned about the detrimental effects of smoking through her school health program. She has told her parents that she wants them to stop smoking because she loves them and wants them to live for a long, long time. Her parents know that it will be tough to stop, but they have enrolled in a community stop smoking program. They have asked adults who visit their home not to smoke. They have put up a no smoking sign by the front door. They are trying to reduce their risk.*

Christabell's parents have made an extraordinary effort to stop smoking because they learned that their smoking was harming their daughter as well as themselves. The children (and spouses) of smokers are, in a way, involuntary smokers themselves because they have no choice but to breathe air that is contaminated with tobacco smoke. Children of cigarette smokers have far more lung illnesses, such as bronchitis and pneumonia, than do children of nonsmoking parents. When Christabell's parents stopped smoking their risk for heart attack was reduced almost immediately, and their daughter's risk of illness was also reduced. Education programs such as Smoke Free Class of 2000 and the American Heart Association School Site Programs can make a real difference for children and their parents. Life insurance companies, rigorous judges of risk, insure nonsmokers and former smokers at substantially lower rates than smokers.

A healthy diet

Parents think a great deal about diet. They know that children need varied and interesting meals, and they often feel overwhelmed by the barrage of advice they receive. Dialogue such as "Eat it up! It's good for you" "But Mom, I *hate* it. It's yucky" can be heard in all families. Constant battling over eating destroys the happy sense of sharing and love that should accompany a family meal. For parents who want to make their children's diet both healthy and enjoyable, these are the important points:

- Start *early*. Young children actually *like* a heart-healthy diet.
- *Involve* the child. Talk about healthful foods. Emphasize the positive; for example, that a lean and healthy person may excel in sports. But avoid emphasis on thinness as a stylish symbol.
- Be *consistent*. Provide heart-healthy foods every day, but don't be a drag. Allow for occasional sprees at birthday parties or other special occasions.
- Set a good *example*.

Remember that as a parent, you are instilling in your children values for a lifetime. Just as you provide moral and ethical guidelines for your child, so, too, you are setting the guidelines for a heart-healthy life style. Healthy diet and exercise are not only good for your child but will improve your chances of enjoying your grandchildren!

The recommendations of the American Heart Association's "prudent diet" are good for the well-being of the entire family. It is important to note also that no modification of the infant-feeding recommendations of the American Academy of Pediatrics—particularly no "low-fat diet"—is advisable for a child under two years of age. Infancy is a time of rapid brain growth, when fats are essential to the development of a normal brain and nervous system.

These are the elements of a heart-healthy diet:

- Keep cholesterol intake low (less than 250 milligrams per day for an adult; limit children to 100 milligrams per one thousand calories).
- No more than 30 percent of calories should come from fats (the average U.S. diet has 40 percent or more).
- The ratio of unsaturated to saturated fat should be at least as high as two to one (saturated fat should be less than 10 percent of calories).
- Carbohydrates, including fresh fruits and vegetables, should compose at least 55 percent of total calorie intake, with complex carbohydrates such as grains and cereals emphasized.
- Proteins should compose 10 to 20 percent of calorie intake, with fish and chicken as the principal protein sources.
- Adults should consume no more than two grams of salt per day; no salt should be added to children's food.

Cholesterol and triglycerides. Cholesterol is an essential part of animal cells. Because cholesterol is manufactured in the liver, even people who have no cholesterol at all in their diet have normal blood levels of cholesterol. On average, 70 percent of our cholesterol is manufactured by our bodies and 30 percent is absorbed from the animal foods that we eat, including eggs, meat, butter, and whole milk.

Cholesterol carried in the blood is attached to proteins known as **lipoproteins.** The **low-density lipoproteins** (LDLs) are sometimes called "bad cholesterol," because high levels of LDL and atherosclerosis go together (the principal protein in LDL is apo B; *apo* means that the protein can attach itself to fats or **lipids**). *High-density lipoproteins* (HDLs), which carry much less cholesterol, are known as "good cholesterol" because high levels appear to be a protection against atherosclerosis. (HDL carries cholesterol from the artery lining back to the liver, where it is broken down and disposed of. The principal protein in HDL is apo A1.)

Triglycerides, fats containing three fatty acids, are present naturally in the body itself, including the bloodstream, and also in food. Although they are less directly involved in causing atherosclerosis than is cholesterol, normal triglycerides are a good sign that the body can handle fats well. Triglycerides in the blood are carried on very-low-density lipoproteins.

In a newborn infant the cholesterol level in the blood is around 150 mg/dl; this level shows little change throughout childhood. A level above 200 mg/dl at any time during childhood is statistically abnormal—95 percent of all children have lower levels—and may be a red flag, a warning to review diet and other risk factors carefully. (Dr. Peter Kwiterovich of Johns Hopkins and other experts recommend these "desirable" levels of cholesterol for children from 2 to 19 years: total cholesterol below 170 mg/dl; LDL cholesterol below 110 mg/dl; HDL cholesterol above 45 mg/dl.) However, cholesterol levels can vary with age, diet, and the child's posture (whether the test is drawn with the child sitting or lying down). Therefore, a single cholesterol level does not establish risk. High levels should be rechecked, and if they are persistently elevated, a lipid profile should be performed. If a child's total cholesterol is 170 mg/dl or higher on the first nonfasting test, a further study should be done after twelve hours of fasting (nothing to eat or drink except water or clear juices); a blood sample obtained from the forearm vein should be tested for LDL, HDL, and triglycerides. With this lipid profile, the pediatrician or practitioner can help the family decide whether any diet precautions are needed, or whether referral to a lipid specialist is the right course.

Should all children have their cholesterol checked?

The answer is a qualified yes. It seems reasonable to check cholesterol in all families with a higher than normal aggregate risk for early coronary artery disease. However, there are several unanswered questions that prevent a blanket recommendation. First, we do not yet know the best time for checking cholesterol in a child. Second, we do not know what numbers are too high. Still, for some families, reassurance that their child's cholesterol is normal is important in its own right.

At present, cholesterol checks are usually recommended around 3 years of age, at 10 to 11 years, and at 18. At least one detailed study of total cholesterol, lipoproteins, and triglycerides is recommended for all children by the time they are ten or eleven. The family's pediatrician should be consulted about where such tests are to be done; a reliable laboratory is essential. Total cholesterol can be measured with only a prick of a finger, and the child need not fast. If this test is normal, and if both parents have normal cholesterol levels, more detailed tests will not be needed on any regular basis. Only if there are special risk factors are more frequent checks indicated.

Recently the National Institutes of Health advised all adults to have periodic cholesterol checks to identify those at increased risk for heart attack, those who need to pay particular attention to diet, and those who may need cholesterol-lowering medication. But general cholesterol testing for all persons, including children, remains a controversial topic. Although experts agree that the origins of atherosclerosis are in childhood, they disagree about the best ways to identify those who are at particular risk. Some suggest testing all children for elevated cholesterol, and this strategy would be effective if childhood cholesterol levels were good predictors of cholesterol levels in adulthood; unfortunately, however, we do not have all the information we need. Studies of a population of children in Muscatine, Iowa, suggest that the future risk of large numbers of children may be misclassified if it is based on cholesterol levels measured in the elementary and middle-school years. One in four boys and almost one in two girls in the Muscatine study who had high cholesterol as children did not have high cholesterol at age twenty. On the other hand, some who had normal cholesterol in childhood had elevated cholesterol when they became young adults. The Muscatine data have put into question the wisdom of generalized testing.

Clearly, a well thought-out national policy on how to approach this complex question of general testing is essential. (The recently published recommendations of the National Cholesterol Education Panel of the National Institutes of Health were used in preparing this chapter.)

The testing of children in high-risk families is on a sounder footing. We know that children of early heart attack victims have marked elevation in total cholesterol and reduced HDL cholesterol. A male child in one of these families already has two risk factors and therefore needs to be particularly conscious of his health and diet.

> *Peter's cholesterol was fine two weeks ago, and now it's 173. That's higher than his grandmother's. What am I going to do?*

What should Peter's mother do about his cholesterol level? First, she should read an authoritative reference, such as *Beyond Cholesterol*, to help her look at the total family history and to give her a balanced view of risk factors. Second, she needs to talk with a good physician with a special interest in heart health (in this case Peter's own pediatrician fills the bill very well). She needs reassurance so she can get away from a preoccupation with cholesterol and back to broader concepts of heart health.

My father had a heart attack when he was only 45. Should I take my daughter Samantha to a lipid clinic?

Families with a history of developing atherosclerosis at an unusually young age do need specialized advice from a family-oriented lipid center to help decide which family members, if any, need medications and changes in diet. Other, rarer, types of familial cholesterol problems exist and help should be sought if there is a family history of early heart attacks.

Familial hypercholesterolemia. Familial hypercholesterolemia is sometimes called *hyper-beta-lipoproteinemia* because the beta or LDL level in the blood is abnormally high. In such cases there is a genetic defect in the receptors of liver and other cells that use cholesterol; as a result of this defect cholesterol is not continually recycled in the body as it should be, but accumulates in the blood and in body tissues. About 1 in 500 of all children do carry one defective gene for this disorder. Children with one defective gene (heterozygotes) have half the normal number of LDL receptors, and the LDL levels in their blood are two to three times the normal levels. Those rare children—about one in a million—who receive an abnormal gene from both parents (homozygotes) have very few receptors, and their LDL blood levels are six to ten times the normal levels. Diet alone is effective in some children who have one defective gene, but many need medication and careful monitoring of the whole family in a specialized lipid clinic. All children who have two defective genes (one from each parent) need specialized care because of the extremely high risk of severe atherosclerosis before the age of twenty.

Blood pressure

Blood pressure problems are rare in childhood. But because high blood pressure levels in a child or adolescent may become dangerous hypertension in an adult, the American Academy of Pediatrics recommends yearly blood pressure checks in children over 3 years old. These pressure readings can then be compared with normal levels for the age (arranged in percentile curves similar to those used for height and weight). Measurements above the 90th percentile, after rechecking, will call for careful watching; measurements above the 95th percentile may require investigation and treatment.

Some families have a strong predisposition to high blood pressure, and children in these families may have blood pressure levels that "track" above the normal range from the early teens. In such children particular attention to salt intake and to maintaining normal weight may help avoid the necessity of taking antihypertensive medications. If no one in the family has a heavy hand with the salt shaker, and if family food shopping is done with awareness of the high salt contents of many convenience foods, the child's salt intake will be adequate and he or she will have the best chance of avoiding hypertension as an adult. There is increasing evidence that regular exercise tends to keep blood pressure levels in the normal range.

Regular physical activity

Some ongoing exercise is beneficial for everyone. You do not need to be a marathon runner to benefit from the cardiovascular effects of physical activity! For adults, even lawn-raking reduces the risk of an early heart attack, and a brisk walk for a half hour a day is nearly as helpful to heart health as running thirty to forty miles each week.

The problem is, how do we get our children to develop the habit of exercise? This generation is the second to be raised in front of a television set and few of our children know the joys of outdoor childhood play—sledding, tag, or kick-the-can. The demands of two-career families, intensive schoolwork, and organized (sometimes overorganized) sports activities at school or in Little League leave little time for families to learn how to exercise together and to prepare for life-long activity.

Prescribing exercise in a way that ensures a child's participation and enjoyment is not easy. Children should be encouraged to find good non-team or solo sports, such as tennis, swimming, bowling, bicycling, and hiking, that can provide exercise throughout their lives. The traditional team competitive sports—football, soccer, baseball, and basketball—are rarely carried on beyond college age. In addition, fewer than 5 percent of high school boys and an even smaller percentage of girls actually participate on the varsity teams. Many boys find that a sport like karate increases their self-confidence and muscle strength; with a good instructor, it can provide excellent regular exercise. Many girls also enjoy learning self-defense. Some children enjoy fencing or dance classes. One does not have to sign up for karate or join a health club to benefit from exercise. It is often worthwhile for a family and its physician to review the family's exercise pattern. If the parents jog or walk or bicycle regularly, usually the children will want to join in. On the other hand, if the parents' weekend exercise consists mostly of trips to the store or the refrigerator, their children may well follow in their footsteps. Fishing trips, volleyball, and swimming are all sports a family can enjoy together.

Heart-Healthy and Heart-Unhealthy Family Lifestyles

Despite the barrage of publicity about heart health, families still differ widely in their awareness of the subject.

A heart-unhealthy family

Harry, who is 11 years old, starts his day with a breakfast of waffles, syrup, and butter accompanied by two glasses of whole milk. He takes to school a packed lunch of salami and mayonnaise on white bread, and adds to it by buying two chocolate bars.

Harry moves around as little as possible during physical education. His teacher does not protest; the school has concluded at various conferences that Harry and his family are "not motivated." After school he watches television until the family goes out for fast food. Harry orders two cheeseburgers, a double order of French fries, and a chocolate sundae. His parents order similar meals. Both of his parents are stout and smoke during the meal. When the weekend comes there is a grand cookout of hot dogs and hamburgers. One of the neighbors tries to start a softball game but Harry's family isn't interested.

On Monday evening Harry goes with his mother to the pediatrician, Dr. C., a slender and active young woman with an athletic family of her own. When Harry's mother says, "Do you think Harry is getting too heavy?" Dr. C. looks at Harry's growth chart. It confirms that Harry's height is average (at the 50th percentile) for his age of 10 years, but that his weight is far above the 95th percentile. "Yes, he's much too heavy. You can see that from the chart. Did I give you a diet sheet last time?" Harry's mother replies, "He just won't stick to his diet. I really tried." Dr. C. admonishes them both and they go home to begin a new week with more of the same behavior.

In the past an overweight child like Harry, with overweight parents, often received little help from a health team. Recently some special clinics have had considerable success in changing unhealthy family patterns. Harry and his family need to be referred to such a group, in which dietary counselling and positive reinforcement replace the old fatalistic attitude "Fat runs in the family." Even when unspoken, this attitude of disapproval and helplessness seems to undermine heart health.

A recent study of overweight adults has shown clearly that certain enzymes may differ in obese and lean persons. Regaining weight once lost, therefore, is much easier for a person who is overweight. Although we do not yet know how much childhood obesity is genetically programmed, we do know that losing weight and maintaining normal weight do not grow easier as time passes. It is hard now, but it will be harder later, so it is better to begin as soon as possible.

> *What's wrong with Harry's hamburger and chocolate sundae diet? My father ate hamburgers and French fries all his life. He died last month at 88 years old. And he loved salt! What about him?*
>
> *Every time you turn on TV, something else is bad for you. I think it's gone too far. My family is going to enjoy their food and not jog themselves to death. Anyway, not all doctors believe in cholesterol, do they?*

It is true that some people can ignore heart-healthy habits and live to a healthy old age. Someone has referred to this pattern as the "Winston Churchill syndrome," a poor and denigrating way to perpetuate the name of one the great men of this century. It is true that some people live as they please and thrive, but for most of us average persons good health, long life, and good health habits go together.

The chief problem is HABIT. Harry is building up habits of consuming excess calories, fats, and sugar—habits that will be hard to break later. The Framingham study, innumerable analyses correlating national eating patterns with rates of heart attack in those countries, and many studies of animals that have been fed high-fat diets all confirm that a diet like Harry's will slowly silt up and pollute his coronary arteries as the years go by. Harry, like all of us and our children, deserves better.

A heart-healthy family

> *Hattie has been on a prudent diet since 3 years of age. Now, at 10 years, she drinks skim milk and eats raw carrots as part of her packed lunch. She plays actively on the playground during physical education and at recess. At home, when her mother bakes cookies, she helps while they discuss how to make the cookies low in fat and sugar but delicious all the same.*

Hattie and her brother Tom join Dad and Mom when they shop for the family groceries, and both participate in helping to plan the family's weekly menu. They learn by doing, reinforcing lessons learned in school. On the weekend Hattie bikes in the local park with her parents and a friend and swims in the local pool. At her checkup the pediatrician finds that Hattie is a little above average for height (60th percentile) and at the 25th percentile for weight.

Getting the child involved

Even at the kindergarten level children are interested in food. It is easy to talk naturally to young children about what foods are both good and appetizing, why regular exercise will help them feel more vigorous, and why smoking, for example, is dangerous. As children grow they become more interested in the circulation and in human ecology. By the time they are 10 no one should be discussing weight or diet in their presence while ignoring *the child*. Children cannot prescribe or fully understand their own needs, but they have to be involved with their own heart and health.

No one on a heart-healthy diet need be deprived of an occasional indulgence. An occasional hot dog, pizza, or ice cream sundae can't hurt. A rigid diet can actually be damaging. A child will not grow normally with *no* saturated fat, for example. And a compulsive focus on diet and exercise can precipitate serious eating disorders such as bulimia or anorexia nervosa.

Preventive Cardiology: The Health Team

All of the above principles involve not only the family but others involved in the health of the growing child, including the pediatrician, teachers, the school nurse, and often the physical education instructor and school guidance counselor. It is difficult to exaggerate the importance of the school in the maintenance of a child's heart health. The family and school working together can greatly improve the outlook for long-term heart health.

The school

The school can help educate the child about a healthy heart. Many biology teachers give excellent courses on the heart and the body's circulation, as we have found from discussions with them and with their pupils. Nature classes and classes in health and biology can be similarly useful. So can field trips to museums that have walk-through hearts, such as the Franklin Museum in Philadelphia, or to embryology laboratories. Such a laboratory may be part of a medical school division of pediatric cardiology or a division of anatomy where research is being done on early development of the chicken heart. The young child, looking through the microscope at the yolk sac of a chicken embryo in a Petri dish, can see the beginning of the heartbeat. Some enterprising biology teachers arrange a special visit to a laboratory for such a demonstration. Long before he has heard of Leonardo da Vinci the young child can share the artist's joy in how the circulation begins.

Physical education teachers can emphasize and encourage each child's natural love of play and activity. We have been lucky in knowing several teachers who have instilled enthusiasm and a life-long dedication to good exercise habits in students with no potential to become star athletes.

The school can also provide heart-healthy meals and snacks. Unfortunately, school lunches are still often high in calories and fat, but in a recent visit to the Baltimore County school system we saw how a good nutritionist can help a school provide food that is nutritious as well as appetizing and popular.

Perhaps most important, the concept of human ecology can be instilled in children. Just as they learn how to preserve and improve the natural environment, so they can learn to preserve and improve their individual health. This topic, of course, is wider than heart health alone.

The physician and the nurse clinician

The doctor who cares for children is concerned with the preservation of health, not merely with the treatment of disease. As the child's friend and advocate, the doctor will monitor blood pressure and cholesterol levels and review the details of diet with as much interest as he or she has in the timing of immunizations. The physician often helps the family by detecting early signs of obesity and by modifying risk factors, nurse-clinicians, active in some medical practices and in clinics, can provide a source of continued practical knowledge and encouragement.

Government and volunteer agencies

Public agencies such as the National Institutes of Health and private agencies such as the American Heart Association can provide many excellent pamphlets and other materials for a family's study. Two booklets the whole family will enjoy are *Children and Smoking: A Message to*

Parents and *Cholesterol and Your Heart*, which provides useful tables on the fat and cholesterol content of certain foods.

Local branches of the American Heart Association often hold meetings on the maintenance of heart health for families, teachers, and dietitians. In Maryland the American Heart Association sponsors a highly successful annual meeting, the Toby Edward Keenan Symposium, which includes sessions for dietitians, teachers, school nurses, and parents on new strategies for heart health. In the 1990 program, which was attended by more than 200 people, the speakers and discussion group leaders were teachers, a school lunch program coordinator, an exercise physiologist, and a cholesterol expert. Such meetings not only update the participants' knowledge but also serve to give substance to the health team concept, the important idea that all of us, in various ways, are working on the same side for the same cause: Keeping a Healthy Heart.

The media, including the major television networks, keep diet and exercise constantly in the news. Some of the energy and ingenuity of their programmers could be put to good use in making heart health a specific topic of interest to families as a whole, to "children of all ages."

The cost to our society from early coronary artery disease is staggering emotionally, medically, and financially. The benefits of reducing atherosclerosis and its health care burden can be even greater.

The challenge of maintaining a healthy child's heart was once confined to the parents of children born with normal hearts. But now that so many heart problems can be treated successfully in early infancy this challenge is also real for parents of children with repaired heart defects. A baby born today with a serious defect such as transposition of the great arteries will have this defect repaired before he or she is a week old. Early follow-up is so encouraging that it seems likely such a child will live a normal life span; therefore, long-term heart health is relevant to such a child.

A healthy heart is a treasure most of us have at birth. Keeping it healthy is a need, a duty, and a vital challenge for each of us and for our children. Even a child born with a heart defect, after successful treatment, can gain a healthy heart and learn to maintain it. The principles are the same for us all.

The Heart of a Child in the Twenty-first Century

In the next century even more children will be born with healthy hearts. Heart defects will become rarer as the environment improves and as more is known about exposure of the unborn to toxins. It is possible, for example, that some families are predisposed to a specific defect but that abnormal development occurs only if the mother or father is exposed to a toxic agent acting through a genetic mechanism. Planning for a healthy baby, then, can in the future be done with the new knowledge that is coming from research. These trends can be expected:

- Worldwide abolition of rheumatic heart disease is entirely feasible. The successful grassroots campaign to abolish smallpox is an example of the extraordinary achievements possible in prevention.

- Cardiomyopathies will yield only as the basic cause of each type is identified, and as a basis for prevention or treatment at the cellular level is discovered. This will be a slow process.

- Although the treatment of arrhythmias will become increasingly reliable and specific, prevention will have to await more understanding of exactly what abnormality in the muscle cell causes the "misfiring" that is the hallmark of severely disordered rhythm. Arrhythmias caused by self-administered toxins such as cocaine should disappear.

- The burden of atherosclerosis on the adult heart has already grown less severe and deaths from coronary disease in young adults have declined. They will decline further.

- The future is bright for countless children born with congenital defects of the heart.

- Collaborative studies and new means of imparting findings will help spread knowledge about heart defects quickly and effectively.

- Studies of families and their genetic makeup will lead to understanding of the genes responsible for the formation of the heart and identification of the gene abnormalities that lead to some heart defects.

- Advances in genetics will lead to strategies to repair some gene defects.

- Research into the true needs of families and children with heart problems will lighten the present burden of care many now experience.

- Increased knowledge of what substances can damage the developing heart will gradually lead to heart health for all children.

Physicians and scientists have developed treatments and strategies that allow even children with many severe defects to live much longer and with a higher quality of life than was possible fifty years ago. The next fifty years will see continued remarkable advances in clinical care and progress in the fundamental understanding of how defects occur in the developing heart. Environmental changes and gene therapy hold the promise of prevention of a host of congenital and acquired health abnormalities. Dedicated teams of physicians, cardiovascular scientists, heart professionals, teachers, and parents will continue to work together to strengthen the hearts of children. The children themselves will learn how to have healthy hearts.

There are several ways of thinking about the impact of childhood heart problems on society, and how this impact might be changed in the next century. One way is to think of the years of potential life lost because of deaths from congenital heart defects. The Centers for Disease Control calculated that in 1970–72, heart defects accounted for 418,134 years of life lost before age 65; by 1984 this figure had fallen to 302,759 years, reflecting the great advances in treatment during the previous decade. As surgical and other treatment advances continue to be made, this premature loss of life will continue to be reduced. Even today, a baby born with a single heart defect and two well-functioning ventricles of adequate size has an almost 95-percent chance of achieving healthy adulthood. For babies born with defects in other systems in addition to the heart itself, and babies born with complex heart abnormalities with underdevelopment of a ventricle, the risk of premature death is still at least ten times higher than that for babies with a single heart defect; such babies are much more likely to need multiple operations and many different types of treatment, and as adults they may not be fully healthy. Future research, therefore, will need to focus on these more severe defects, and on how the formation of muscle cells in the embryonic heart interacts with the formation of the walls and the valves of the heart. In the past, when deaths from all types of heart defects were frequent, it was difficult to see that such heart defects have a spectrum of severity; with the extraordinary treatment advances of the twentieth century, the concept of the spectrum of severity becomes important as a focus for future research. Much work will be required to learn exactly how and why the more severe defects occur, and how the chances of normal heart development can be increased in such children.

Throughout this book, we have explained that *all* heart abnormalities begin in the young, many before birth, even though the abnormality may be silent in childhood and not recognized until adult years. The most important example, statistically, of such unrecognized problems is coronary heart disease, which accounts for eight to ten times as many years of lost productive life as congenital heart defects do. In preventive cardiology we study how to decrease the risk factors for atherosclerosis in later life, beginning in childhood. Research is slowly and laboriously building our knowledge of how the genes that control cholesterol interact with diet and other environmental changes to cause the present high (though improving) rate of coronary atherosclerosis in the Western world. There is something a little scary about some of this new knowledge—we will soon be able to predict, for example, when we look at a healthy newborn baby with completely normal coronary arteries, what the chances will be that he or she will develop colon cancer, Huntington's chorea, heart attack, or other diseases. Yet, at the same time, it is encouraging that in almost all diseases the risk can be reduced by healthy living.

The study of the physical change over time in response to genes and to environmental change is known as *developmental biology*. Although we all stop growing in height at a certain age, usually around 18 to 20 years, our bodies and our hearts continue to change all of our lives. It is essential that we discover how we change and why if disease is to be controlled. Like atherosclerosis, cardiomyopathy, for example, has both genetic and environmental causes; prevention of the abnormality can occur only when these causes are identified.

Beginning in 1978, three international symposia on the development of the heart have been held in Tokyo. The 1989 symposium emphasized molecular biology techniques as a means of understanding how genes influence heart growth, how the various proteins in the heart muscle differ in health and in disease, and how tissues from outside the heart itself, such as the neural crest cells, may move into the heart as it forms. Other studies have focused on the effect of increases in heart rate or blood pressure on the growth and formation of the heart. The proteins of the heart muscle and the growth factors that regulate the timing of action of heart genes are also beginning to be understood.

Advances such as these in knowledge of the development of the heart will continue over the years; they will have enormous impact on our lives and the lives of children not yet born. When the heart of a child is healthy, we must do all we can to keep it so. If it is badly formed or unhealthy, we must help to find the best treatment. Treatment is not just a mechanical process, but an interaction between child, family, and health team to restore and preserve one of life's great wonders, the healthy heart of a child.

Appendix:
Groups That Can Help

Family support groups can be a source of comfort, information, and friendship. One family support group in Maryland, Big Hearts for Little Hearts, can be reached through the Division of Pediatric Cardiology at the Johns Hopkins Hospital, 600 N. Wolfe Street, Baltimore, Maryland 21205. In the Rochester, New York, area, contact Helping Hearts, Division of Pediatric Cardiology, Box 631, University of Rochester Medical Center, Rochester, New York 14642.

A list of local family support groups can be obtained from the local affiliate of the American Heart Association (check the business pages of the telephone book) or by writing to the Council of Cardiovascular Disease in the Young, American Heart Association, National Center, 7320 Greenville Avenue, Dallas, Texas 75231. The American Heart Association will also provide booklets about specific topics on request.

Glossary

Acidosis: The accumulation of acid products in the blood after either a severe episode of oxygen lack or failure of the circulation.

Acquired heart disease: A heart problem that is not due to a congenital defect, but that appears or is acquired after birth, such as rheumatic heart disease or myocarditis.

Aneurysm: A ballooning out of the wall of an artery or vein or of the heart wall due to weakening of the wall by injury or disease or to some abnormality dating from birth.

Angina pectoris: Chest pain due to heart disease. A condition in which the heart muscle doesn't receive enough blood, usually due to coronary insufficiency.

Angiocardiography: An X-ray examination of the blood vessels or chambers of the heart. A special fluid (called "contrast material" or "dye"), visible to X-ray, is injected into the bloodstream. Also called *angiography*; the X-ray pictures made are called *angiograms*. *Cineangiography* is the recording of angiograms on cinefilm.

Angioplasty: A procedure sometimes used to dilate (widen) narrowed arteries. A catheter with a deflated balloon on its tip is passed into the narrowed artery segment, the balloon inflated, and the narrowed segment widened.

Aorta: The large artery that receives blood from the heart's left ventricle and distributes it to the body.

Aortic valve: The heart valve between the left ventricle and the aorta. It normally has three flaps, or cusps; when only two cusps are present the valve is said to be "bicuspid."

Aphasia: The inability to speak, write, or understand spoken or written language because of brain injury or disease.

Arrhythmia (or **dysrhythmia**): An abnormal rhythm of the heart.

Arteriography: A testing procedure, similar to angiography, in which an X-ray-opaque dye is injected into the bloodstream and pictures of arteries (usually the coronary arteries) are taken and studied to see if the arteries are damaged.

Arterioles: Small, muscular branches of arteries. When they contract, they increase resistance to blood flow, and blood pressure in the arteries increases.

Arteriosclerosis: Commonly called "hardening of the arteries," the term refers to a variety of conditions that cause artery walls to thicken and lose elasticity.

Artery: Any one of a series of blood vessels that carry blood from the heart to the various parts of the body. Arteries have thick, elastic walls that can expand as blood flows through them.

Atherosclerosis: A form of arteriosclerosis in which the inner layers of artery walls become thick and irregular due to deposits of fat, cholesterol, and other substances. These deposits, sometimes called "plaques," cause the arteries to narrow and the flow of blood through them is reduced.

Atresia: A complete failure of development of a structure normally present and open at birth, as in pulmonary valve atresia (affecting the heart), or intestinal atresia (affecting part of the intestine).

Atria (singular, **atrium**): The two upper holding chambers of the heart. The right atrium receives blood from the body; the left atrium receives blood returning from the lungs via the pulmonary veins.

Atrial septal defect: A congenital defect in the atrial septum. Most defects are in the middle part of the septum (*ostium secundum defect*); some are in the upper part of the septum, often with abnormal drainage of the right pulmonary veins (*sinus venosus defect*). A defect low in the atrial septum with an abnormal mitral valve, a form of endocardial cushion defect, is sometimes referred to as an *ostium primum*.

Atrial septum: The wall or septum dividing the right from the left atrium.

Atrioventricular (AV) node: A small mass of specialized conducting tissue at the bottom of the right atrium through which the electrical impulse stimulating the heart to contract must pass to reach the ventricles.

Atrioventricular canal defect (also *endocardial cushion defect* or *atrioventricular septal defect*): A congenital defect in which the mitral and tricuspid valves are abnormal and defects are present between the atria and ventricles. Large defects are called "complete atrioventricular canal defects." "Incomplete" or partial defects, including

ostium primum, affect mostly the atrial septum and are less severe.

Atrium: See **atria**.

Bacterial endocarditis: A bacterial infection of the heart lining or valves. It occurs more often in people with abnormal heart valves or congenital heart defects than in those with normal hearts. Bacterial endocarditis prophylaxis (**BE prophylaxis**) means precautions taken to prevent endocarditis.

Balloon catheter: A specialized catheter used to dilate a narrowed structure in the circulation: See **angioplasty** and **valvuloplasty**.

Blood pressure: The force or pressure exerted by the heart in pumping blood; the pressure of blood in the arteries.

Blue babies: Babies who have a blue tinge to their skin (cyanosis) resulting from insufficient oxygen in the arterial blood; this blue color often indicates a heart defect.

Bradycardia: Slow heart rate.

Bronchial arteries: See **collateral circulation**.

Capillaries: Microscopically small blood vessels between arteries and veins that distribute oxygenated blood to the body's tissues.

Cardiac: Pertaining to the heart.

Cardiac arrest: Cessation of the heartbeat.

Cardiac catheterization: The process of examining the heart by introducing a thin tube (catheter) into a vein or artery and passing it into the heart.

Cardiac jelly: A substance found early in heart development that helps to form the framework on which the heart valves are formed.

Cardiology: The study of the heart and its functions in health and disease.

Cardiomyopathy: A disorder of the muscle of the heart.

Cardiopulmonary resuscitation (CPR): A technique combining chest compression and mouth-to-mouth breathing, used during cardiac arrest to keep oxygenated blood circulating in the body.

Cardiovascular: Concerning the heart and blood vessels.

Cerebral embolism: A blood clot formed in one part of the body and then carried by the bloodstream to the brain, where it lodges in an artery.

Cerebral thrombosis: Formation of a blood clot in an artery that supplies part of the brain.

Cholesterol: A fat-like substance manufactured in the body and found in foods from animal sources, such as whole-milk dairy products, meat, fish, poultry, animal fats, and egg yolks.

Cineangiogram: See **cineangiography**.

Cineangiography (also called *cineangiocardiography*): The technique of taking moving pictures, known as **cineangiograms**, to show the passage of an X-ray opaque dye through blood vessels.

Circulatory system: System comprising the heart and blood vessels, responsible for the circulation of the blood.

Closed-heart surgery: Surgery that does not require the heart-lung machine and is performed on blood vessels in the chest but outside the heart itself.

Clot (also **blood clot**): A jelly-like mass of blood tissue formed by clotting factors in the blood. Clots stop the flow of blood from an injury. Clots also can form inside an artery whose walls are damaged by atherosclerotic buildup and can cause a heart attack or stroke.

Coarctation: Narrowing of the aorta where the pulmonary artery and aorta are joined by the ductus arteriosus.

Collateral circulation: A system of smaller arteries, closed under normal circumstances, that may open up and start to carry blood to part of the heart when a coronary artery is blocked. These arteries can serve as alternate routes of blood supply. Collateral vessels in the lungs (bronchial arteries) may be found in severely blue (cyanotic) children.

Complex heart defects: Abnormalities of the heart in which there are several defects, so that one of the ventricles or pumping chambers has failed to develop; or in which a major artery or heart valve is completely blocked (atretic). Children with such defects usually need several operations.

Computerized axial tomography (CAT) scan: A specialized X-ray technique producing a three-dimensional image using a rotating X-ray beam.

Congenital: Refers to conditions existing at birth.

Congenital heart defect: Malformation of the heart or its major blood vessels present at birth.

Congestive heart failure: See **heart failure**.

Conotruncal area: The part of the heart joining the right ventricle to the pulmonary artery. If the conotruncal area does not develop normally, blood flow between heart and lungs is disturbed and blueness or cyanosis occurs.

Coronary arteries: Two arteries arising from the aorta that arch down over the top of the heart, branch, and provide blood to the heart muscle.

Coronary artery disease: Conditions that cause narrowing of the coronary arteries so blood flow to the heart muscle is reduced.

Coronary bypass surgery: Surgery to improve blood supply to the heart muscle.

Coronary thrombosis: Formation of a clot in one of the arteries that conduct blood to the heart muscle. Also called *coronary occlusion.*

Cyanosis: Blueness of the skin and body tissues caused by insufficient oxygen in the blood.

Defibrillator: An electronic device that helps reestablish normal contraction rhythms in a malfunctioning heart.

Diabetes (also **diabetes mellitus**): A disease in which the body doesn't produce or properly use insulin. Insulin is a hormone that the body needs to convert sugar and starch into the energy needed in daily life.

Diastole: The time when the ventricles, the pumping chambers of the heart, relax and receive blood from the atria, the receiving chambers.

Diastolic blood pressure: The lowest blood pressure measured in the arteries, measured when the heart muscle is relaxed between beats.

Digitalis (also **digoxin, digitoxin**): A drug that strengthens the contraction of the heart muscle, slows the rate of contraction of the heart, and promotes the elimination of fluid from body tissues. Digitalis is often used to treat heart failure and also to treat certain arrhythmias.

Diuretic: A drug that increases the rate at which urine forms by promoting the excretion of water and salts.

Doppler-echocardiography: See **echocardiography**.

Doppler shift: A sound, such as the sound of a siren or train whistle, increases in pitch as it approaches and decreases as it moves away. This change in pitch or frequency, the Doppler shift, is used to calculate the speed or velocity of the source of sound and sound waves.

Ductus arteriosus: An artery present before birth that connects the aorta and pulmonary artery. The ductus normally closes shortly after birth; if it remains open (**patent ductus arteriosus**), medical or surgical treatment may be necessary.

Echocardiography: A diagnostic method in which pulses of sound are transmitted into the body and the echoes returning from the surfaces of the heart and other structures are electronically plotted and recorded. In Doppler-echocardiography the speed with which the waves travel can be measured, allowing for measurements of pressure changes across the heart valves. Doppler color flow mapping superimposes color on the image received back from the heart; this color is useful in showing the direction of blood flow across valves or through small defects in the heart, which might otherwise be difficult to detect.

Echo-Doppler: See **echocardiography.**

Edema: Swelling due to an abnormally large amount of fluid in body tissues.

Elective referral: A nonemergency consultation about a heart murmur or other medical problem.

Electrocardiogram (EKG): A graphic record of electrical impulses produced by the heart.

Electroencephalogram (EEG): A graphic record of the electrical impulses produced by the brain.

Electrophysiologic study (EPS): A detailed, highly specialized study of the conducting system of the heart performed in the cardiac catheterization laboratory.

Embolus: A blood clot that forms in a blood vessel in one part of the body and then is carried to another part of the body.

Endocardial cushions: Formed in part from the cardiac jelly, the cushions form the infrastructure for the developing valves of the heart.

Endocardium: The smooth inner lining of the heart wall, lying between the heart muscle (myocardium) and the blood inside the heart chambers.

Endothelium: The smooth inner lining of many body structures, including the heart and blood vessels.

Enzyme: A complex organic substance capable of speeding up specific biochemical processes in the body.

Exercise testing: A study of how much exercise an individual can do compared to others of the same age and size with normal hearts; the test is done using either a treadmill or a stationary bicycle, while the EKG, blood pressure, and breathing are monitored.

Extrasystole: An extra heartbeat, a form of arrhythmia, usually not needing treatment.

Fetal Doppler-echocardiography: A detailed examination of the baby's heart while the baby is still in the mother's womb. This test may be done in a specialized center (in addition to the usual ultrasound tests for the baby's growth), if there is any reason to suspect an abnormality of the rhythm or structure of the developing heart.

Fibrillation (also **atrial** or **ventricular fibrillation**): Rapid, uncoordinated contractions of individual heart muscle fibers. The heart chamber involved can't contract all at once and pumps blood ineffectively, if at all.

Fibrin: A protein in the blood that enmeshes blood cells and other substances during blood clotting.

Foramen ovale: A small opening in the atrial septum present before birth.

Gradient: A change in pressure across a heart valve or between different heart chambers.

Health team: The group of professionals helping the child and the family achieve heart health.

Heart attack: Death of or damage to an area of the heart muscle due to a reduced supply of blood to that area. Also *myocardial infarction, coronary occlusion.*

Heart block: When the heartbeat does not pass normally from the atrium to the ventricles, heart block is present. This is a form of abnormal heart rhythm (arrhythmia).

Heart failure: The inability of the heart to pump out all the blood that returns to it. This failure results in a backup of blood in the veins that lead to the heart and sometimes an accumulation of fluid in the lungs and various parts of the body.

Heart-lung machine: An apparatus that oxygenates and pumps blood while a person's heart is opened for open-heart surgery.

Heredity: The genetic transmission of a particular quality or trait from parent to offspring.

Heterotaxy: Abnormal arrangement of the heart and the abdominal organs, often with multiple defects in the heart and absent or multiple spleens.

High blood pressure: A chronic increase in blood pressure above its normal range.

High-density lipoprotein (HDL): A carrier of cholesterol believed to transport cholesterol away from the tissues to the liver, where it can be excreted.

Holter monitoring (ambulatory electrocardiography): The EKG is recorded on tape over twenty-four to seventy-two hours, then analyzed for arrhythmias or other abnormalities.

Hypertension: High blood pressure.

Hypoplastic: Too small or poorly developed. In the most severe heart flow defects, either the right or the left ventricle may be hypoplastic and incapable of functioning normally.

Hypoxia: Too low a level of oxygen in the blood and tissues of the body.

Incidence: The number of new cases of a disease that develop in a population during a specified period of time, such as a year.

Interrupted aortic arch: An extreme form of **coarctation** of the aorta.

Invasive: Entering the body. Cardiac catheterization and angiography are sometimes called "invasive" procedures, because a catheter is introduced into the body through a vein or artery. By contrast, echocardiography or magnetic resonance imaging are described as "noninvasive," because nothing is introduced into the body.

Ischemia: Decreased blood flow to an organ, usually due to constriction or obstruction of an artery.

Ischemic heart disease: Also called *coronary artery disease* and *coronary heart disease*. This term is applied to heart ailments that are caused by narrowing of the coronary arteries and that therefore are characterized by a decreased blood supply to the heart.

Kawasaki disease (syndrome): An acute illness of children characterized by fever, rash, swelling, and inflammation of various parts of the body. The coronary arteries or other parts of the heart are affected in 20 percent of children with this disease.

Left-heart flow defect: A congenital abnormality affecting the ventricle or the valves and arteries on the left side of the heart, due to abnormal flow patterns during embryonic life.

Lipid: A fatty substance insoluble in blood.

Lipoprotein: A lipid surrounded by a protein; the protein makes it soluble in the blood.

Looping: Looping of the heart, so that the heart apex points to the left, occurs early in development; when the process is abnormal a cardiac looping defect occurs.

Low-density lipoprotein (LDL): The main carrier of harmful cholesterol in the blood.

Lumen: The opening of a tube, such as a blood vessel.

Magnetic resonance imaging (MRI) (also called *nuclear magnetic resonance*): An imaging method using radio frequency pulses in a magnetic field to define body structures.

Mitral valve: The heart valve between the left atrium and left ventricle. It has two flaps, or cusps.

Mucocutaneous lymph node syndrome: See **Kawasaki disease**.

Murmur (heart murmur): An extra sound between the two normal heart sounds "lub" and "dup." Most murmurs in children are innocent, but some indicate a heart problem needing treatment.

Myocardial infarction: See **heart attack.**

Myocardium: The muscular wall of the heart that contracts to pump blood out of the heart and relaxes when the heart refills with returning blood.

Obesity: The condition of being significantly overweight.

Open-heart surgery: Surgery performed on the opened heart while the bloodstream is diverted through a heart-lung machine. Also called *cardiopulmonary bypass surgery.*

Ostium primum defect: See **Atrial septal defect.**

Oximetry (pulse oximetry): A technique for measuring the oxygen saturation in the blood.

Pacemaker or **sinus (sinoatrial) node**: A small mass of specialized cells in the right atrium of the heart that produces the electrical impulses that cause contractions of the heart. The term "artificial pacemaker" is applied to an electrical device that can substitute for a defective natural pacemaker and control the beating of the heart by transmitting a series of rhythmical electrical discharges.

Pericarditis: Inflammation of the pericardium.

Pericardium: The membrane forming the outer lining of the heart, separating the myocardium, or heart muscle, from the lungs and other structures in the chest.

Platelets: One of three kinds of formed elements found in the blood. Platelets aid in the clotting of the blood.

Pulmonary: Pertaining to the lungs.

Pulmonary artery: The artery carrying blood from the heart to the lungs.

Pulmonary atresia: Failure of development of the pulmonary valve or the pulmonary artery.

Pulmonary blood flow: The flow of blood into the lungs with each heartbeat. The amount of flow depends on the size of the child, increasing with age. It is normally equal to the flow of blood to the body (systemic blood flow).

Pulmonary valve: The valve between the right ventricle and the pulmonary artery. The pulmonary valve, like the aortic valve, opens and closes with each heartbeat. The valve usually has three leaflets or cusps; when two leaflets are present the pulmonary valve is said to be "bicuspid."

Rheumatic heart disease: Damage done to the heart, particularly to the heart valves, by one or more attacks of rheumatic fever.

Right-heart flow defect: A congenital abnormality of the ventricle, or the valves and arteries on the right side of the heart, due to abnormal flow patterns during embryonic life.

Rubella: A viral illness, commonly known as German measles, that causes fever and a rash. When a woman develops rubella during her first three months of pregnancy, the exposed baby may be born with heart defects and other problems.

Septation: The process of development of the septa of the heart, resulting in the four separate chambers of the normal newborn heart.

Septum (plural **septa**): The wall dividing the heart chambers into right and left sides. The atrial septum separates the right from the left atrium; the ventricular septum separates the two ventricles.

Stenosis: Narrowing or obstruction of a valve or opening, which may be present from birth (as in pulmonary valve stenosis) or follow rheumatic heart disease (as in mitral stenosis).

Streptococcal infection: A bacterial infection, usually in the throat, resulting from the presence of an unusual form of streptococcus.

Syndrome: A combination of problems or defects often seen together. See chapter 14 for a listing of some syndromes with heart involvement.

Systemic blood flow: The flow of blood to the body with each heartbeat. The amount of flow increases as the child grows.

Systole: The time when the ventricles contract and pump blood out to the body and the lungs.

Systolic blood pressure: The highest blood pressure measured in the arteries, measured when the ventricle is contracting and pumping blood to the body during systole.

Tachycardia: Fast heart rate.

Tetralogy of Fallot: A conotruncal heart defect with a large ventricular septal defect and pulmonary stenosis, leading to cyanosis.

Thrombosis: The formation or presence of a blood clot (thrombus) inside a blood vessel or cavity of the heart.

Tricuspid atresia: Failure of development of the tricuspid valve, associated with a hypoplastic right ventricle.

Truncus arteriosus: A conotruncal defect in which a single artery or trunk leaves the heart, due to a failure of the normal embryonic division of the truncus into the aorta and pulmonary artery.

Valvuloplasty: Dilation of a narrowed valve using a **balloon catheter.**

Vascular: Pertaining to the blood vessels.

Vein: Any one of the vessels of the vascular system that carry blood from various parts of the body back to the heart.

Ventricle: One of the two lower (pumping) chambers of the heart. The left ventricle pumps blood to the body, the right ventricle to the lungs.

Ventricular hypertrophy: Thickening (*hyper*, too much; *troph*, growth) of the muscle forming the wall of the ventricle. Ventricular hypertrophy is usually a response to some obstruction in the heart or blood vessels, but is sometimes part of a heart muscle disease (cardiomyopathy).

Ventricular septal defect: See **ventricular septum.**

Ventricular septum: The wall separating the right from the left ventricle. If the wall is incomplete, a ventricular septal defect is present; the defect may lie in the upper part of the wall (membranous or perimembranous defect) or lower down the wall, in the muscular ventricular septum.

Viral myocarditis: Inflammation of the myocardium with a virus; this inflammation sometimes leads to a chronic disease of the heart muscle, cardiomyopathy.

Further Reading

J. Burn. "The Aetiology of Congenital Heart Disease." In *Paediatric Cardiology*, ed. R. H. Anderson, F. J. Macartney, E. A. Shinebourne, and M. Tynan. Vol. 1. Edinburgh: Churchill Livingstone, 1987. (This chapter contains an excellent review of syndromes with heart involvement.)

Edward B. Clark and Atsuyoshi Takao, eds. *Developmental Cardiology: Morphogenesis and Function*. Mount Kisco, N.Y.: Futura, 1990.

George Howe Colt. "Last Chance for Baby Dylan." *Reader's Digest* 137 (October 1990): 83–88.

C. Ferencz. "Epidemiology of Congenital Heart Disease. The Baltimore-Washington Infant Study 1981–1989." In *Perspectives in Pediatric Cardiology*, ed. R. H. Anderson. Mt. Kisco, N.Y.: Futura, 1993.

C. Ferencz and A. Correa Villasenov. "Epidemiology of Cardiovascular Malformations: The State of the Art. *Cardiology in the Young* 1 (1991): 264–284.

Lyn Frederickson. *Confronting Mitral Valve Prolapse Syndrome*. San Marcos, Calif.: Avant Books, 1989.

Arthur Garson, Jr., J. T. Bricker, and D. G. McNamara, eds. *The Science and Practice of Pediatric Cardiology*. Philadelphia: Lea & Febiger, 1990. (Chapter 34, "Basic Aspects of Doppler Echocardiography," by Daniel J. Murphy, Jr., contains a good description of the scientific basis of the use of this technique in children and adults.)

J. W. Kirklin. "The Movement of Cardiac Surgery to the Very Young." In *Perspectives in Pediatric Cardiology*, ed. G. Crupi, L. Parenzan, R. H. Anderson. Vol. 2. Mt. Kisco, N.Y.: Futura, 1989. (This is a summary of recent progress by one of the masters of surgery.)

Peter Kwiterovich. *Beyond Cholesterol: The Johns Hopkins Complete Guide for Avoiding Heart Disease*. Baltimore: Johns Hopkins University Press, 1989.

Thomas K. Miller and Jayne M. Miller. *Baby James: A Legacy of Love and Family Courage*. New York: Harper, 1988.

J. H. Moller, W. A. Neal, and W. Hoffman. *A Parents' Guide to Heart Disorders*. Minneapolis: University of Minnesota Press, 1988.

J. H. Moller, C. Patton, R. L. Varco, and C. W. Lillehei. "Late results (30 to 35 years) after Operative Closure of Isolated Ventricular Septal Defect from 1954 to 1960." *American Journal of Cardiology* 68 (1991): 1491–1497.

D. Naylor, T. J. Coates, and J. Kan. "Reducing Stress in Pediatric Cardiac Catheterization." *American Journal of Diseases in Children* 138 (1984): 726–729.

Catherine A. Neill. "Quality of Life Issues in the Adult with Congenital Heart Disease." *Quality of Life and Cardiovascular Care* 3 (1987): 5–14.

———. "Quality of Life Issues in the Adult with Congenital Heart Disease, Part II: The Next Generation." *Quality of Life and Cardiovascular Care* 3 (1987): 57–64.

M. K. Park, ed. *Pediatric Cardiology for Practitioners*, 2d ed. Chicago: Mosby Year Book, 1988.

John Stone. "Chest Pains: What Do They Mean?" *New York Times Magazine*, 19 February 1989.

Karen Stray-Gundersen, ed. *Babies with Down Syndrome: A New Parents' Guide*. Rockville, Md.: Woodbine House, 1986.

V. T. Thomas. *Pioneering Research in Surgical Shock in Cardiovascular Surgery: Vivien Thomas and His Work with Alfred Blalock*. Philadelphia: University of Pennsylvania Press, 1985.

Lorraine M. Wright and Maureen M. Leahey, eds. *Families and Chronic Illness*. Springhouse, Pa.: Springhouse, 1987.

Index

The Heart of a Child

Designed by Ann Walston

Composed by Brushwood Graphics, Inc.
in ITC Berkeley Oldstyle

Printed by The Maple Press Company
on 50-lb. Glatfelter Eggshell Cream
and Bound in Holliston Aqualite